HYPERTENSION AND
CO-EXISTING DISEASE

Hypertension and Co-existing Disease

FRANCISCO LEYVA MD MRCP

Consultant Cardiologist
Good Hope Hospital
Sutton Coldfield
Birmingham, UK

ANDREW COATS FRCP DM FESC FACC

Professor of Cardiology
Department of Cardiac Medicine
National Heart and Lung Institute
Imperial College School of Medicine
Royal Brompton and Harefield NHS Trust
London, UK

Blackwell Science

© 2000 by
Blackwell Science Ltd
Editorial Offices:
Osney Mead, Oxford OX2 0EL
25 John Street, London WC1N 2BL
23 Ainslie Place, Edinburgh EH3 6AJ
350 Main Street, Malden
    MA 02148-5018, USA
54 University Street, Carlton
    Victoria 3053, Australia
10, rue Casimir Delavigne
    75006 Paris, France

Other Editorial Offices:
Blackwell Wissenschafts-Verlag GmbH
    Kurfürstendamm 57
    10707 Berlin, Germany

Blackwell Science KK
    MG Kodenmacho Building
    7–10 Kodenmacho Nihombashi
    Chuo-ku, Tokyo 104, Japan

First published 2000

Set by Graphicraft Limited, Hong Kong
Printed and bound in Great Britain at
MPG Books Ltd, Bodmin, Cornwall

DISTRIBUTORS

    Marston Book Services Ltd
    PO Box 269
    Abingdon, Oxon OX14 4YN
    (*Orders*: Tel: 01235 465500
                Fax: 01235 465555)
USA
    Blackwell Science, Inc.
    Commerce Place
    350 Main Street
    Malden, MA 02148-5018
    (*Orders*: Tel: 800 759 6102
                     781 388 8250
                Fax: 781 388 8255)
Canada
    Login Brothers Book Company
    324 Saulteaux Crescent
    Winnipeg, Manitoba R3J 3T2
    (*Orders*: Tel: 204 837-2987)

Australia
    Blackwell Science Pty Ltd
    54 University Street
    Carlton, Victoria 3053
    (*Orders*: Tel: 3 9347 0300
                Fax: 3 9347 5001)

A catalogue record for this title
is available from the British Library and
the Library of Congress

ISBN 0-632-05073-X

The Blackwell Science logo is a
trade mark of Blackwell Science Ltd,
registered at the United Kingdom
Trade Marks Registry

For further information on
Blackwell Science, visit our website:
www.blackwell-science.com

Contents

Preface

Where does a doctor go for advice when investigating or managing a patient? Frequently to a senior colleague or to a local expert opinion. Doctors rarely consult textbooks for routine management decisions. Is this because time is too precious or is it because the conventional format of a textbook with its chapters on epidemiology, pathology, presenting features and therapeutics is not tuned to the needs of the busy clinician? In practice, patients present with problems, framed against their personal characteristics, co-morbidity and expectations. What the doctor managing individual patients needs is a quick access guide to specialist advice framed in such a way that it can be directly applied to individual patients. We have tried to devise a novel textbook of hypertension, one which is practical in every sense; it is framed with the contexts of clinical practice in mind. It presents lists of options and advice points, not for memorization, but as checklists and solutions. The format takes the doctor through possible patient types and possible clinical scenarios, heavily cross-referenced so that the physician can deal with a second or third issue that arises during the discussion. We hope the doctor will quickly find a solution, which may be 'best available' when no strictly evidence-based answer exists.

In the last few years there have been several developments which are likely to have a major impact on clinical practice in the millennium. Firstly, diagnostic and treatment options have proliferated at breathtaking speed, and with this so has the complexity of choosing the best approach for each patient. Secondly, the wider society has increased expectations of medicines and the medical community. It expects more but is increasingly less tolerant of errors or omissions. The medical profession no longer can justify doing its collective best if that means using clinical opinions formed during training which may now be out of date. Lastly, there has been a profusion of guidelines to aid doctors in their practice, partially in response to the first two pressures. These are usually written by experts but often after extensive deletions of any recommendations that could be challenged in any aspect. The guidelines develop in a way that ensures they are opinion-free tomes with every statement carefully backed up by trial evidence and carefully worded so as to offer no offence to any influential medical opinion. As a result they are often bland, conservative and of little value in real clinical situations. Unfortunately, despite major advances in clinical trial evidence in cardiovascular medicine, there remains the bulk of clinical practice which cannot be based solely on the results of randomized controlled trials. In the setting of clinical practice, every patient is unique and presents unique problems. The issues of practice can, however, be addressed by analogy to a limited number of clinical settings.

We have written this text as a way of condensing the clinical evidence together with our own practice opinions in a way which is both accessible and comprehensive and which will aid in the practical management of patients with high blood pressure. Almost all patients and clinical scenarios will be accessed at least approximately by the clinical settings of the chapters. We have for this reason introduced unusual chapters for a textbook on hypertension, highlighting common medical settings for advice such as hypertension in women, stroke prevention, hypertension complicated by cardiac disease, and hypertension in the setting of other cardiovascular risk factors such as dyslipidaemias, diabetes and insulin resistance. The chapters and sections on drug treatments offer real practical advice on when to choose certain agents.

Like housework, best medical practice is never finished, and we as authors would value your opinions on areas not covered, on problems not addressed and on issues that remain difficult or controversial. Should time and energy allow a revision, we consider such feedback to be the essential component for ensuring we continue to meet the needs of the doctor managing patients with hypertension.

F. Leyva
A.J.S. Coats
London

Abbreviations

ACE	angiotensin-converting enzyme
ACTH	adrenocorticotrophic hormone
AER	albumin excretion rate
AF	atrial fibrillation
AME	apparent mineralocorticoid excess
BMI	body mass index
CABG	coronary artery bypass grafting
CHD	coronary heart disease
CK	creatine kinase
DHA	docosahexaenoic acid
DTPA	diethylenetriamine penta-acetic acid
ECG	electrocardiograph
EDTA	ethylenediamine tetra-acetic acid
EF	ejection fraction
EPA	eicosapentaenoic acid
ESR	erythrocyte sedimentation rate
GFR	glomerular filtration rate
GTN	glyceryl trinitrate
HDL	high-density lipoprotein
HMG-CoA	3-hydroxy-3-methylglutaryl coenzyme A
HRT	hormone replacement therapy
IDDM	insulin-dependent diabetes mellitus
IDL	intermediate-density lipoprotein
INR	international normalized ratio
ISA	intrinsic sympathomimetic activity
ISH	International Society of Hypertension
JVP	jugular venous pressure
LDL	low-density lipoprotein
LVH	left ventricular hypertrophy
MAOI	monoamine oxidase inhibitor
MI	myocardial infarction
MR	mitral regurgitation
NIDDM	non-insulin-dependent diabetes mellitus

NSAID	non-steroidal anti-inflammatory drug
SIADH	syndrome of inappropriate antidiuretic hormone
TIA	transient ischaemic attack
VLDL	very low-density lipoprotein
WHO	World Health Organisation

Part 1 Diagnosis

1: Blood Pressure Measurement

Since Hales' demonstration that blood pressure could be measured using a glass tube inserted into an artery of a horse, numerous devices have been used for the measurement of blood pressure in humans. In 1896, Riva-Rocci devised a clinically applicable sphygmomanometer and a method for measurement using arterial occlusion. This technique was later modified by Korotkoff who, in 1905, introduced a technique for measuring systolic and diastolic blood pressure.

A century later, blood pressure is the most frequently measured clinical variable in hospital and general practice. Because hypertension is an incurable condition that will affect patients for life, its measurement becomes of paramount importance. Numerous techniques are now available for its measurement. Whilst intra-arterial measurement is the scientific gold standard, sphygmomanometry has been the technique adopted by all the large epidemiological studies and clinical outcome trials of antihypertensive therapy. As a consequence, current definitions of hypertension and management guidelines are all based on measurements derived from the Korotkoff technique and the mercury sphygmomanometer.

MERCURY SPHYGMOMANOMETRY

Numerous reviews [1,2], reports of expert committees [3,4] and practical guides [5,6] have been published on the subject. In terms of accuracy and reliability, the mercury sphygmomanometer (Fig. 1.1) is superior to other devices, including the aneroid variety. Detection of auscultatory sounds (Table 1.1; Fig. 1.2) using the Riva-Rocci/Korotkoff method is the most appropriate technique in most clinical settings. The steps in the measurement of blood pressure using mercury sphygmomanometry are as follows:

• Place the sphygmomanometer no further than 1 m from the observer, with the mercury column in the vertical position and at eye level (reading the meniscus at an angle will result in errors).

• Ideally, ensure that the patient has fasted for at least 2 h (blood pressure falls postprandially, particularly in the elderly) and has refrained from

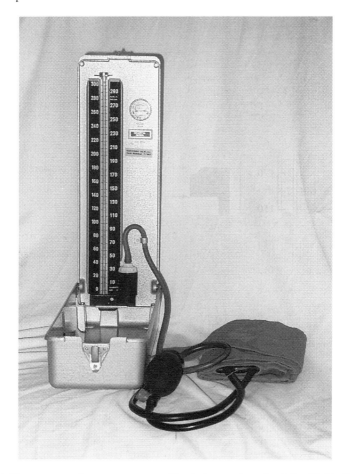

Figure 1.1 The mercury sphygmomanometer. The device consists of an inflatable bladder covered by a cuff of inelastic cloth, a rubber bulb which acts as the pump, airtight rubber tubing and a mercury manometer. The minimum length of tubing between the cuff and the manometer should be 70 cm and of the tube between the inflation source and the cuff 30 cm. All connections should be airtight and the tubing should be checked regularly for cracks. The mercury and glass column should be kept clean and periodic checks should be made to ensure that the mercury meniscus is visible at zero. The bladder length and width should be at least 80% and 40% of the arm circumference (at the midpoint of the arm), respectively. Some cuffs are equipped with markers to help avoid miscuffing. Some have a marker for positioning accurately over the brachial artery. Bladder undersizing is more common than oversizing. Undersizing with too short or too narrow a bladder will cause overestimation of blood pressure; oversizing with too wide or too long a bladder will cause underestimation. Composites of three inflatable bladders are available, but they have not been satisfactorily evaluated.

smoking or ingesting caffeine within 30 min before measurement. Ask the patient to rest for at least 5 min.
• At the time of measurement, ask the patient to sit upright and comfortably. The whole arm should be uncovered, supported, and positioned at the level

Table 1.1 Brachial artery sounds during sphygmomanometry.

Phase I	First appearance of repetitive, tapping sounds, taken as the **systolic pressure**
Phase II	Tapping sounds take a softer, swishing quality
Phase III	Tapping sounds return. Their intensity may exceed that of phase I sounds
Phase IV	Muffling of sounds, which gradually become softer in quality
Phase V	Point at which all sounds disappear, taken as the **diastolic pressure**

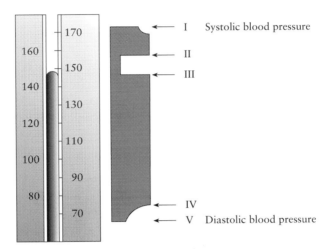

Figure 1.2 In blood pressure measurement, a note should be made as to the presence of an auscultatory gap, which occurs in individuals in whom phase I sounds disappear and then reappear as the arm cuff is deflated. If the systolic pressure is not palpated, one may erroneously take the systolic pressure as the point at which the phase I sounds appear for the second time. The auscultatory gap is frequently present in the elderly and in pregnant women. Taking phase IV as the diastolic blood pressure is acceptable in situations where sounds persist much beyond muffling. Both phase IV and phase V pressure should be noted in pregnancy. Reproduced with permission from L. Hansson *et al. Clinician's Manual on Hypertension* 1990, p. 11. Science Press Ltd, London.

of the heart (midsternum), holding the patient's arm at the elbow. The patient's legs should be uncrossed.

- Select an appropriate cuff size (Table 1.2), ensuring that the bladder encircles at least two-thirds of the arm. Wrap the cuff around the arm so that its centre, or marker, overlies the brachial artery and its lower edge is about 3 cm above the elbow crease.
- Place the tubing at the upper side of the cuff or on the posterior aspect of the arm, so as not to interfere with auscultation.
- To minimize anxiety, warn the patient that there will be minor discomfort when the cuff is inflated.
- Determine the position of the brachial pulse.

Table 1.2 Recommended bladder sizes.

	Width (cm)	Length (cm)
Children	12	18
Small child	4	13
Young child	8	18
Most adults (standard)	12	26
Obese adults	12	40

Adapted with permission from [5].

- To measure *systolic blood pressure*:
  - Keep palpating the brachial pulse, over the area of strongest pulsation. Tighten the valve and inflate the cuff rapidly to 30 mmHg above the palpated systolic pressure.
  - Place the diaphragm of the stethoscope over the brachial pulse, securing it by pressing lightly on the bell with the thumb and ensuring that nothing else is touching the stethoscope.
  - Then, deflate slowly ($\approx$ 2 mm s^{-1}) by loosening the valve until faint, repetitive, tapping sounds first appear. This point (phase I) should be taken as the systolic blood pressure.
- To measure *diastolic blood pressure*:
  - Continue to deflate the cuff slowly until all sounds disappear completely. This so-called phase V should ordinarily be taken as the diastolic blood pressure.

Although this method provides highly accurate results, care must be taken to minimize false-positive and false-negative results, i.e. recording a blood pressure that is not representative of the patient's mean blood pressure (Table 1.3). On documenting measurements, the following items should be considered:
- Measurements of systolic and diastolic blood pressure should not be rounded off to the nearest 5 or 10 mmHg, but to the nearest 2 mmHg.
- At the first visit, blood pressure should be recorded in both arms and the highest reading recorded. In 10% of the elderly, blood pressures differ by > 10 mmHg between the arms.
- Two or more readings should be averaged; if the first two differ by more than 5 mmHg, additional readings should be obtained in the same session.
- A note should be made as to whether or not the patient was nervous during blood pressure measurement.
- A note should be made as to the presence of an auscultatory gap. This gap occurs in individuals in whom phase I sounds disappear and then reappear as the arm cuff is deflated. If the systolic pressure is not palpated, one may erroneously take the systolic pressure as the point at which the phase I sounds

Table 1.3 Sources of errors in measuring blood pressure using sphygmomanometry.

Instrument	Faulty manometer
	Pressure leaks (esp. from cracked rubber tubing)
	Faulty stethoscope
	Inadequately sized bladders:
	Undersizing, variation of up to 12/8 mmHg; up to 30 mmHg in obesity
	Oversizing, variation in the range of 10–30 mmHg
	Limited accuracy of the device
Observer	Systematic errors
	Hearing problems
	Inconsistency in recording sounds
	Reading the mercury meniscus at an angle
	Terminal digit preference (numbers ending in 0, 5, odd or even numbers)
	Bias towards preconceived 'normal' blood pressures
Patient	White-coat effect*
	Posture (lying, standing, sitting)
	Respiration
	Poor arm support†
	Arm position in relation to the heart‡
	Anxiety and restlessness§
	Diurnal variation
	Food intake
	Tobacco
	Alcohol
	Body temperature
	Bladder distension
	Exercise
	Pain

*May contribute to up to 30 mmHg.
†Diastolic blood pressure may increase by as much as 10% if the arm is extended and unsupported.
‡Can affect blood pressure readings by as much as 10 mmHg [7].
§More frequent in children.
For further details, consult [7].

appear for the second time. The auscultatory gap is frequently present in the elderly and in pregnant women.

• The timing of antihypertensive drug intake prior to the measurement should be recorded.

SEMI-AUTOMATIC DEVICES (Fig. 1.3)

Semi-automatic devices work on the principle of detection of sounds by a microphone or by detection of arterial blood flow using ultrasonography or oscillometry. Cuffs can be inflated manually or automatically or both. Some devices designed for hospital use can be programmed for measurement at specified time intervals.

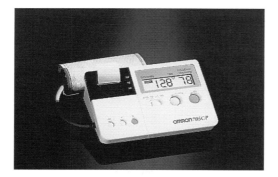

Figure 1.3 The Omron HEM-705CP, a semi-automated device for the self-measurement of blood pressure.

Table 1.4 Validation of semi-automatic devices.

Device fulfilling the BHS protocol for accuracy
Omron HEM-705CP
Devices *not* fulfilling the BHS protocol for accuracy
Omron HEM-400C
Philips HP5306
Philips HP5308
Philips HP5332
Fortec DrMI-100
Systema DrMI-150
Nissei DS-175
Nissei BPM
Healthcheck CX-5

Self-measuring semi-automated devices validated against the British Hypertension Society (BHS) protocol for accuracy by one laboratory over a 5-year period. Reproduced with permission from [5].

The use of semi-automatic devices is increasingly supported by data from clinical trials. For example, in a recent report of the HOT (Hypertension Optimal Treatment) study, measurements taken at home and in the office were comparable, and both measurements were able to separate patients into appropriate target groups for treatment [8]. This study employed a calibrated and validated oscillometric device with digital readout (Visomat OZ, D2 International, Hestia Pharma GmbH).

Although many commercially available semi-automatic devices are inaccurate compared to the mercury sphygmomanometer, some are accurate and reliable (Table 1.4). If they are to be used for home measurement, patients should be advised on which devices have satisfied the accuracy criteria of the British Hypertension Society (BHS) or the American Association for Advancement of Medical Instrumentation (AAMI, on http://www.aami.org).

Table 1.5 Devices which have been shown to fulfil the AAMI and BHS accuracy criteria.

Manufacturer	Device	Mechanism
Disetronic Medical Systems	CH-Druck	Auscultatory
	Prolifomat	Auscultatory
IDT	Nissei DS-240	Auscultatory
		Oscillometric
Welch Allyn	Quiet Track	Auscultatory
SpaceLabs Inc	SpaceLabs 90202	Oscillometric
	SpaceLabs 90207	Oscillometric
A&D Company	TM-2420 Model 6	Auscultatory
	TM-2420 Model 7	Auscultatory
	TM-2421	Oscillometric

The assessment took place in January 1995. AAMI, American Association for the Advancement of Medical Instrumentation; BHS, British Hypertension Society. Reproduced with permission from [9].

The use of wrist and finger blood pressure measuring devices should be discouraged until they are appropriately validated.

AMBULATORY BLOOD PRESSURE MONITORS

Whereas self-monitoring can provide measurements over many days and weeks, ambulatory monitoring provides numerous measurements over prolonged periods, usually 24 h. Technical errors are relatively small compared with errors involved in estimates based on a small number of clinical readings. Such errors can be minimized by calibrating it against a mercury sphygmomanometer immediately before use. Recommended devices are shown in Table 1.5 and in Fig. 1.4.

VALUE OF SELF-MEASUREMENT AND AMBULATORY BLOOD PRESSURE MEASUREMENT

Self-measured blood pressures are highly reproducible [10], accurate [11] and predictive of end-organ damage [12]. Similarly, ambulatory measurements show a closer correlation with end-organ involvement (particularly left ventricular hypertrophy) [13] and are better predictors of morbidity and mortality [14,15] than clinical measurements. Notwithstanding, self-measurement and ambulatory blood pressure monitoring should not be used routinely. They may be helpful when the following are suspected:
• White-coat hypertension;
• Borderline hypertension;
• Episodic hypertension (as in phaeochromocytoma);

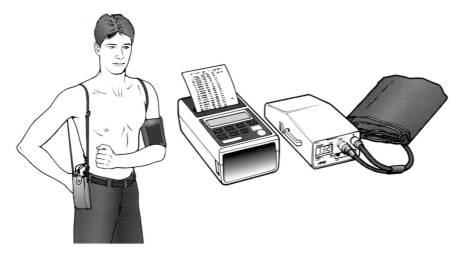

Figure 1.4 An ambulatory blood pressure monitor. The TM2421 blood pressure monitor (supplier: P.M.S. (Instruments) Ltd, Maidenhead, UK) has fulfilled the American Association for the Advancement of Medical Instrumentation and the British Hypertension Society accuracy criteria. The device provides a printed readout. Alternatively, measurements can be fed into a personal computer for further analysis using dedicated software.

- Isolated systolic hypertension;
- Resistant hypertension.

Some authorities advocate the use of ambulatory blood pressure monitoring in the diagnosis and management of hypertension in pregnancy. It should be noted, however, that in pregnancy, there is no established blood pressure threshold on which treatment should be initiated on 24-h ambulatory monitoring and self-monitoring. Typical 24-h profiles in different conditions are shown in Fig. 1.5.

BLOOD PRESSURE MEASUREMENT IN SPECIAL GROUPS

Children

Children present special problems in blood pressure measurement [16]. Blood pressure is much more variable than in adults and, therefore, single measurements are less likely to reflect the child's average blood pressure. Because variability is least with systolic blood pressure, it is this which should be used in diagnosis. Brachial sounds can be difficult to detect in children under 5 years of age and in such cases, oscillometry and Doppler ultrasound may be useful. The choice of cuff is particularly important (Table 1.2).

The elderly

Blood pressure is considerably more variable in the elderly than in the young. Because single measurements are less likely to reflect the individual's average

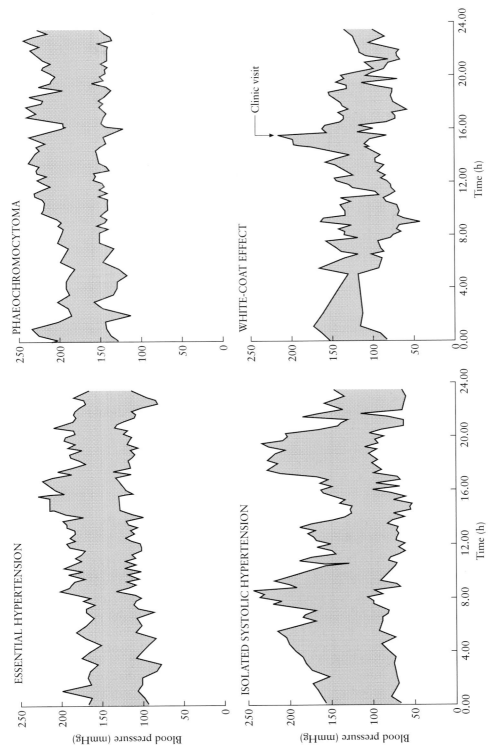

Figure 1.5 Ambulatory blood pressure profiles over 24 h in different situations.

blood pressure, repeated measurement is particularly important. In 10% of elderly patients, blood pressures differ by > 10 mmHg between the arms and therefore, blood pressure should be taken in both arms at the initial visit. Blood pressure measurements in the elderly should not be taken within 2 h after meals, as postprandial blood pressure falls are particularly pronounced.

In the elderly, age-related reductions in arterial wall elasticity and distensibility give rise to a disproportionate rise in systolic blood pressure which may be manifested as isolated systolic hypertension (ISH). Reduced arterial compliance may prevent complete occlusion of the brachial artery during blood pressure measurement and lead to erroneous blood pressure readings (pseudohypertension). Because of the long auscultatory gap that is frequently present, the systolic blood pressure should first be estimated by palpation. Measurement by auscultation should then be taken using an appropriately sized cuff, ensuring that it is then inflated to 30 mmHg above the palpated systolic pressure (page 6).

Pregnancy

The hyperdynamic circulation of pregnancy gives rise to a greater variability in the phase V sound, which may occasionally reach zero. For this reason, some authorities prefer to use the phase IV rather than the phase V sound as the diastolic blood pressure. Against this approach is the fact that the phase IV sound is subject to a more frequent interobserver and intraobserver variability than the phase V sound. Although there is no evidence that one sound is superior to another in predicting end-organ damage, taking the phase IV sound may offer a wider margin of safety. On balance, we suggest that phase IV and V sounds be recorded and that phase IV (muffled sounds) be used for diagnosis.

Blood pressure in pregnancy is heavily dependent on posture. Brachial artery blood pressure is highest with the patient sitting upright, intermediate in the supine position and lowest in the left lateral position.

Measuring blood pressure in pregnancy

- Ask the patient to lay in the left lateral position with a tilt of 30° and the upper arm positioned at the level of the heart
- Measure blood pressure as usual (Chapter 1), recording phase IV and V Korotkoff and using phase IV sounds (muffled sounds) for diagnosis

---

Arrhythmias

Sudden variations in cardiac rhythm lead to sudden changes in cardiac output and, therefore, in blood pressure. Thus, cardiac arrhythmias, such as atrial fibrillation, lead to beat-to-beat variations in systolic and diastolic blood pressure. There is no agreed method for measuring blood pressure using sphygmomanometry in such cases. We would recommend taking the systolic blood pressure as the first appearance of sounds (phase I) and the diastolic blood pressure as the point of final disappearance of all sounds (phase V), ignoring isolated extra beats.

In bradyarrhythmias, deflating the cuff rapidly may result in the sounds being missed, causing underestimation of systolic blood pressure and overestimation of diastolic blood pressure. In this situation, it is advisable to deflate the cuff very slowly, around 1–2 mmHg s^{-1}.

Obesity

The width of the inflatable bladder should be 40% of the circumference of the midpoint of the arm and the length should be 80% of the arm circumference. A cuff with a bladder measuring 12×40 cm should be adequate for most obese adults.

Postural hypotension

This is particularly common in the elderly. It may be caused by all antihypertensive drugs, particularly diuretics and β-blockers, and by other drugs, such as tricyclic antidepressants and neuroleptics. Other causes include autonomic neuropathy, as in diabetes mellitus.

About 20% of elderly individuals have postural falls of > 20 mmHg in systolic blood pressure [17]. Estimation of postural drops should be performed in symptomatic patients and should include measurement of blood pressure after 5 min rest and then after standing for 1–2 min. Checking for postural hypotension in the clinic, however, is often unrewarding. A more formal assessment, using ambulatory blood pressure monitoring or tilt-testing, may be more helpful. By whichever method, the sitting rather than the standing blood pressure should be taken for the purpose of antihypertensive treatment. Ambulatory blood pressure monitoring may be useful when postural drops are not detected in patients presenting with postural symptoms.

The white-coat effect

It has long been recognized that blood pressure measurements taken by patients are about 8/4 mmHg lower than those taken by doctors in the clinic [18–21]. More recently, ambulatory blood pressure monitoring has confirmed that in susceptible non-hypertensive [22] and hypertensive [23] individuals, clinical measurements do not accurately reflect their usual level of blood pressure. This phenomenon, known as white-coat hypertension, carries a favourable prognosis and there is no evidence at present that patients with white-coat hypertension benefit from antihypertensive treatment. Some authorities, however, have suggested that white-coat hypertension may not be entirely innocent, as suggested by reports of its association with functional cardiac abnormalities [24,25] and micro-albuminuria [26]. Others believe that white-coat hypertension is the prelude to hypertension proper.

Estimates of prevalence of white-coat hypertension vary from 20 to 39% [27–29]. It is most readily diagnosed by comparing clinical blood pressures to measurements taken using ambulatory blood pressure monitoring or validated automated self-measuring devices. White-coat hypertension should be considered in:

• Individuals in whom the diagnosis of hypertension is being considered for the first time.

• Individuals who are currently being treated for mild-to-moderate hypertension and who have no hypertensive end-organ damage or associated cardiovascular risk factors.

• Individuals who have not responded as predicted to antihypertensive treatment.

• Individuals who suffer side-effects suggestive of hypertension after initiation of treatment.

No evidence-based recommendations can be made as to how to follow up patients with white-coat hypertension. Until such evidence is available, we currently recommend that such patients should be followed up with ambulatory blood pressure monitoring every 2–3 years. In a case of a confirmed white-coat hypertensive, there is little point in taking further clinical blood pressure measurements.

References

1 Webb CH. The measurement of blood pressure and its interpretation. *Prim Care* 1980; 7: 637–651.

2 Steinfeld L, Alexander H, Cohen ML. Updating sphygmomanometry. *Am J Cardiol* 1974; 33: 107–110.

3 Kirkendall WM, Burton AC, Epstein FH *et al.* Recommendations for human blood pressure determination by sphygmomanometers: report of a subcommittee of the Postgraduate Education Committee, American Heart Association. *Circulation* 1967; 36: 980–988.

4 Frohlich ED, Grim C, Labarthe DR *et al.* Recommendations for human blood pressure determination by sphygmomanometers. *Hypertension* 1988; 11: 209A–221A.

5 O'Brien ET. General principles of blood pressure measurement. In: O'Brien E, Beevers D, Marshall H, eds. *ABC of Hypertension.* London: BMJ Publishing Group, 1995: 3–8.

6 Hill MN. Hypertension: what can go wrong when you measure blood pressure. *Am J Nurs* 1980; 80: 942–946.

7 Kirkendall WM, Feinlieb M, Freis ED *et al.* Recommendations for human blood pressure determination by sphygmomanometers. Subcommittee of the AHA Postgraduate Education Committee. *Circulation* 1980; 62: 1146A–1155A.

8 Kjeldsen SE, Hedner T, Jamerson K *et al.* Hypertension Optimal Treatment (HOT) Study. Home blood pressure in treated hypertensive subjects. *Hypertension* 1998; 31: 1014–1020.

9 O'Brien E. Ambulatory blood pressure measurement. In: O'Brien E, Beevers D, Marshall H, eds. *ABC of Hypertension.* London: BMJ Publishing Group, 1995: 28–34.

10   James GD, Pickering TG, Yee LS *et al.* The reproducibility of average ambulatory, home, and clinic pressures. *Hypertension* 1988; 11: 545–549.

11   Gould BA, Kieso HA, Hornung R *et al.* Assessment of the accuracy and role of self-recorded blood pressure in the management of hypertension. *BMJ* 1982; 285: 1691–1694.

12   Kleinert HD, Harshfield GA, Pickering TG *et al.* What is the value of home blood pressure measurement in patients with mild hypertension? *Hypertension* 1984; 6: 574–578.

13   Verdecchia P, Schillaci G, Boldrini F *et al.* Risk stratification of left ventricular hypertrophy in systemic hypertension using noninvasive ambulatory blood pressure monitoring. *Am J Cardiol* 1990; 66: 583–590.

14   Perloff D, Sokolow M, Cowan R. The prognostic value of ambulatory blood pressure. *JAMA* 1983; 249: 2792–2798.

15   Perloff D, Sokolow M, Cowan R. The prognostic value of ambulatory blood pressure in treated hypertensive patients. *J Hypertens* 1991; 9 (Suppl. 1): S33–S40.

16   Report of the Task Force on Blood Pressure Control in Children. *Pediatrics* 1977; 59 (Suppl.): 797–820.

17   Rutan GH, Hermanson B, Bild DE, Kittner SJ, LaBaw F, Tell GS. Orthostatic hypotension in older adults. The Cardiovascular Health Study. *Hypertension* 1992; 19: 508–519.

18   Sokolow M, Werdegar D, Kain HK *et al.* Relationship between level of blood pressure measured casually and by portable recorders and severity of complications in essential hypertension. *Circulation* 1966; 34: 279–298.

19   Mengden T, Battig B, Edmonds D *et al.* Self-measured blood pressures at home and during consulting hours: are there any differences? *J Hypertens* 1990; 8 (Suppl. 3): S15–S19.

20   Battig B, Steiner A, Jeck T *et al.* Blood pressure self-measurement in normotensive and hypertensive patients. *J Hypertens* 1989; 7 (Suppl. 3): S59–S63.

21   Laughlin KD, Sherrard DJ, Fisher L. Comparison of clinic and home blood pressure levels in essential hypertension and variables associated with clinic home differences. *J Chronic Dis* 1980; 33: 197–206.

22   Floras JS. Will knowing the variability of ambulatory blood pressure improve clinical outcome? An additional consideration in the critical evaluation of this technology. *Clin Invest Med* 1991; 14: 231–240.

23   Mancia G, Sega R, Milesi C, Cesana G, Zanchetti A. Blood pressure control in the hypertensive population. *Lancet* 1997; 118: 867–882.

24   Glen SK, Elliot HL, Curzio JL, Lees KR, Reid JL. White-coat hypertension as a cause of cardiovascular dysfunction. *Lancet* 1996; 348: 654–657.

25   Kuwajima I, Sozuki Y, Fujisawa A, Kjuramoto K. Is white-coat hypertension innocent? Structure and function of the heart in the elderly. *Hypertension* 1993; 22: 826–831.

26   Hoegholm A, Bang LE, Kristensen KS, Nielsen JW, Holm J. Microalbuminuria in 411 untreated individuals with established hypertension, white-coat hypertension, and normotension. *Hypertension* 1994; 24: 101–105.

27   Krakoff LR, Elson H, Phillips RH *et al.* Effect of ambulatory pressure monitoring on the diagnosis and cost of treatment for mild hypertension. *Am Heart J* 1988; 116: 1152–1154.

28   Lerman CE, Brody DS, Hui T *et al.* The white-coat hypertension response: prevalence and predictors. *J Gen Intern Med* 1989; 4: 225–231.

29   Pickering TG, James GD, Boddie C *et al.* How common is white-coat hypertension? *JAMA* 1988; 259: 225–228.

2: Clinical Assessment

HISTORY

The diagnosis of hypertension is usually made incidentally or opportunistically at a routine medical examination or at a consultation for another problem. Headaches, epistaxis and other symptoms, although associated with hypertension by patients [1,2], are of no diagnostic value. The only parameter on which the diagnosis of hypertension is made is the level of blood pressure. The history may point to pathogenetically associated disorders, to manifestations of hypertensive end-organ damage or to other factors which are relevant to management.

Past medical history
Patients should specifically be asked about the following:
- Coronary heart disease (CHD) — angina or myocardial infarction (MI);
- Diabetes mellitus;
- Stroke and transient ischaemic attacks;
- Peripheral vascular disease;
- Dyslipidaemia;
- Gout;
- Hypertension in pregnancy;
- Ureteric or renal problems in childhood;
- Polycystic kidney disease;
- Polycystic ovary syndrome — oestrogen deficiency is associated with increased CHD risk;
- Hysterectomy/oophorectomy — a premature menopause is associated with an increased CHD risk;
- Menopausal status (date of last menstrual period), given the association between the menopause and increased cardiovascular risk;
- Sexual dysfunction — may influence choice of antihypertensive drug.

Family history
Specific questions should be asked about the following:

Table 2.1 Drugs which are known to increase blood pressure.

Oestrogen-based oral contraceptives
Non-steroidal anti-inflammatory drugs (NSAIDs)
Adrenocorticotrophic hormone (ACTH)
Glucocorticoids
Mineralocorticoids
Anabolic steroids
Liquorice and carbenoxolone
Monoamine oxidase (MAO) inhibitors
Ephedrine
Cyclosporin
Cocaine
Clonidine withdrawal*
Tricyclic antidepressants
Serotonin and noradrenaline reuptake inhibitors

*On clonidine withdrawal, blood pressure returns to pre-treatment levels.

- Early CHD: angina, MI or sudden death;
- Type II diabetes mellitus;
- Stroke and transient ischaemic attacks;
- Peripheral vascular disease;
- Dyslipidaemia, polygenic or familial;
- Polycystic kidney disease (autosomal dominant).

Drug history
Specific questions should be asked about prescribed or unprescribed medications which increase blood pressure (Table 2.1).

Social history
Specific questions should address the following:
- Occupation — may affect choice of antihypertensive drug;
- Smoking, quantified in number of cigarettes/day;
- Alcohol intake, quantified in units in the past week [units of alcohol = (volume of drink in ml × alcohol by volume percentage)/1000; 1 unit = 8 g ethanol = 10 ml by volume of pure ethanol];
- Physical activity.

Review of systems
Special attention should focus on the following:
- Chest pain, palpitations, dyspnoea, peripheral oedema, claudication;
- Visual disturbances, motor deficits, either transient or permanent;
- Haematuria, dysuria, prostatism;
- Menopausal symptoms (Chapter 9).

EXAMINATION

As with the history, the examination in a hypertensive patient is often not fruitful. It may, however, point towards:
• Hypertensive end-organ damage;
• Causes of secondary hypertension;
• Other cardiovascular risk factors;
• Coincidental conditions, pathogenetically related or unrelated to hypertension.

General examination

Obesity. Most authorities recommend measurement of height and weight as part of a screening examination. The body mass index (BMI), which provides a convenient and reliable measure of body fat, is calculated as follows:

BMI = weight (kg)/[height (m)]^2

Although definitions of obesity vary, it is generally accepted that a patient with a BMI of $\geq$ 30 kg m^{-2} should be considered obese. A BMI of < 25 kg m^{-2} is considered normal. In adolescents, a BMI $\geq$ 85th percentile for age and gender should be considered overweight.

Smoking. Nicotine-stained fingers may be evident.

Metabolic/endocrine disorders. Check for the following:
• Hypothyroidism;
• Acromegaly;
• Cushing's syndrome;
• Xanthelasmata and tendon xanthomata;
• Gouty joints — gout is associated with increased CHD risk;
• Porphyria;
• Gordon's syndrome (short stature, hypoplastic incisors; very rare).

Cardiovascular examination

Pulse. No changes in the radial pulse are specific for hypertension. The following features, however, may reflect associated disease:
• Sinus tachycardia — this may be a manifestation of left ventricular dysfunction, either systolic or diastolic. Less commonly, it may be due to hyperthyroidism and, rarely, to phaeochromocytoma.
• Irregularly irregular pulse. This is most often a reflection of atrial fibrillation.
• Low-volume, slow-rising pulse: moderate-to-severe aortic stenosis.
• 'Collapsing' pulse: aortic regurgitation.
• Radiofemoral delay in coarctation of the aorta.

Jugular venous pressure (JVP). No changes in the jugular venous pressure are specific for hypertension. The following features, however, may reflect associated disease:
• Absent pulsations: the normal 'fluttering' character of the jugular vein pulsation is absent in atrial fibrillation.
• Raised JVP — may be found in heart failure secondary to hypertensive left ventricular dysfunction or to a previous MI.

Apex beat. The following features may reflect hypertensive heart damage:
• Forceful ('heaving' or 'thrusting') apex beat — in left ventricular hypertrophy. It may be both forceful and 'sustained' in aortic stenosis.
• The apex beat may be abnormally forceful ('heaving', 'thrusting' or 'sustained') in left ventricular (LV) hypertrophy. Its displacement away from the normal position in the fifth intercostal space, midclavicular line, may occur in cardiac enlargement, be it enlargement of the LV cavity or the LV wall.

Heart sounds and murmurs. The only manifestation of hypertension in the heart sounds may be increased intensity of the aortic component of the second sound, reflecting increased diastolic blood pressure. This, however, can hardly be used as evidence of hypertension. Other heart auscultatory findings, reflecting associated disease, may include:
• *Aortic murmurs.* The most common, particularly in elderly hypertensive patients, will be that of aortic sclerosis, which is of no clinical consequence. In the young, a loud midsystolic murmur may be caused by coarctation of the aorta. If in adults, a midsystolic or 'ejection systolic' murmur is associated with a low-volume, slow-rising pulse and clinical or ECG signs of left ventricular hypertrophy and/or signs of left ventricular enlargement, it is likely to be caused by aortic stenosis (Fig. 2.1), which has important implications in management. An early diastolic murmur may be a result of aortic regurgitation (Fig. 2.2), secondary to hypertension or to the degenerative aortic valve disease which occurs in elderly hypertensive patients. A wide pulse pressure, though frequently quoted in the literature, need not be present in this aortic regurgitation.
• *Mitral murmurs.* Left ventricular distension, be it secondary to hypertension or to previous myocardial infarctions, is associated with dilation of the mitral valve annulus. This leads to a failure of apposition of the mitral valve leaflets and to so-called 'functional' mitral regurgitation (Fig. 2.3).

Peripheral pulses and bruits. At the screening visit, in particular, attention should be focused on peripheral pulses and bruits. Absence or reduced intensity of the pulses or bruits may indicate arterial disease:
• Carotid bruits. The presence of a carotid bruit is a very unreliable sign

Systolic
murmur

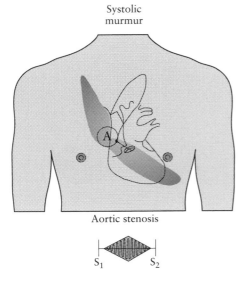

Aortic stenosis

Figure 2.1 Aortic stenosis. The murmur commences immediately after the first heart sound, reaches a peak in midsystole and does not reach the second heart sound. It is best heard with the patient sitting forward on full expiration and radiates to the carotids. Reproduced with permission from B. Erickson. *Guía Práctica de los Latidos y Murmullos del Corazón* 1990. WB Saunders Co., Philadelphia, PA.

Diastolic
murmur

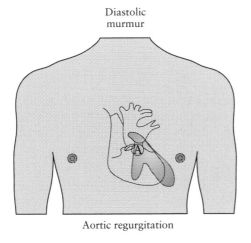

Aortic regurgitation

Figure 2.2 Aortic regurgitation. The murmur of aortic regurgitation reaches its peak in the first third of diastole and wanes in intensity towards mid-diastole. It is best heard at the left sternal edge with the patient sitting forward on full expiration. Reproduced with permission from B. Erickson. *Guía Práctica de los Latidos y Murmullos del Corazón* 1990. WB Saunders Co., Philadelphia, PA.

of the presence or severity of carotid artery disease [3]. Its absence does not exclude carotid disease. Because asymptomatic carotid stenosis is a risk factor for both cardiac events and stroke [4,5], the presence of a carotid bruit and the findings of investigations such as carotid ultrasonography should be taken into account in the assessment of overall cardiovascular risk.

• Femoral bruits, popliteal, posterior tibial and dorsalis pedis pulses may be reduced in volume or may not be palpable in peripheral vascular disease.

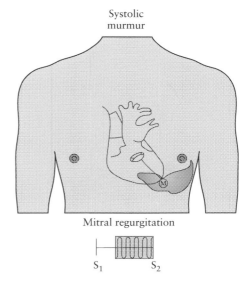

Systolic murmur

Mitral regurgitation

S_1 S_2

Figure 2.3 Mitral regurgitation (MR) produces a high-pitched, blowing pansystolic murmur of constant intensity, best heard at the apex, with radiation to the axilla. It is confined to late systole in mild MR, as in mitral valve prolapse or papillary muscle dysfunction. In severe mitral regurgitation, the murmur superimposes the second heart sound and is therefore described as pansystolic. Reproduced with permission from B. Erickson. *Guía Práctica de los Latidos y Murmullos del Corazón* 1990. WB Saunders Co., Philadelphia, PA.

- Epigastric (renal artery) bruits may be present in patients with renal artery stenosis, but they are by no means a specific sign. The finding of a lateralized bruit which continues into diastole is particularly suggestive.

Respiratory examination
Check for the following:
- Pulmonary crepitations may be present if there is pulmonary oedema. It is noteworthy that in hypertensive patients, heart failure can occur even before there is clinically evident cardiomegaly. The association of a resting tachycardia and pulmonary crepitations in a hypertensive patient should be investigated further (chest X-ray and/or echocardiogram) (see Chapter 5).
- Hyperexpansion and wheezing may be present in coincidental chronic obstructive airways disease.
- Kyphoscoliosis may be present in coincidental osteoporosis, common in postmenopausal women. It may also cause aortic regurgitation.

Abdominal examination
Check for the following:
- Hepatomegaly may reflect associated alcoholic liver disease.
- Expansile aortic pulsation may reflect an abdominal aortic aneurysm — a finding which would make the presence of renal artery stenosis more likely.
- Ballotable kidneys may be present in polycystic kidney disease.

Neurological examination
This may reveal evidence of a previous stroke. Neurogenic causes of hypertension should also be considered (Chapter 10).

Examination of the eyes

External examination may reveal an arcus, suggesting underlying hyperlipi-daemia. Ophthalmoscopy may reveal evidence of:
- Hypertensive retinal disease, including focal arteriolar constrictions, arteriovenous 'nipping', haemorrhages, exudates and papilloedema;
- Diabetic retinopathy;
- Retinal vein or retinal artery occlusion.

References

1   Bulpitt CH, Fletcher AE. Importance of well-being to hypertensive patients. *Am J Med* 1988; 84 (Suppl. 1B): 40–46.
2   Weiss NS. Relation of high blood pressure to headaches, epistaxis and selected other symptoms. *N Engl J Med* 1972; 287: 631–633.
3   Davies KN, Humphrey PRD. Do carotid bruits predict disease of the internal carotid artery? *Postgrad Med J* 1994; 70: 433–435.
4   Norris JW, Zhu CZ, Bornstein NM, Chambers BR. Vascular risks of asymptomatic carotid stenosis. *Stroke* 1991; 22: 1485–1490.
5   Hennerici M, Hülsbömer H-B, Hefter H, Lammerts D, Rautenberg W. Natural history of asymptomatic extracranial arterial disease. Results of a long-term prospective study. *Brain* 1987; 110: 777–791.

3: Investigation of Essential Hypertension

The diagnosis of hypertension is made on the basis of blood pressure levels on repeated measurement. As with the clinical history and examination, the purpose of investigating patients with hypertension is to identify the following:
- Hypertensive end-organ damage;
- Causes of secondary hypertension;
- Other cardiovascular risk factors;
- Coincidental conditions, pathogenetically related or unrelated to hypertension.

A number of routine investigations should be carried out on all patients in whom the diagnosis of hypertension has been confirmed on clinical assessment. Abnormalities which emerge from the clinical assessment and routine investigations should guide further, targeted investigations (Fig. 3.1).

ROUTINE INVESTIGATIONS

All patients who are confirmed hypertensive should have a number of routine investigations (Table 3.1). All are readily available in both hospital and general practice.

Full blood count
This is a complementary investigation which is unlikely to help in the diagnosis of the causes or effects of hypertension. Anaemia (normocytic/normochromic) may be present in chronic renal failure. Polycythaemia may suggest an underlying renal carcinoma or obstructive airways disease.

Erythrocyte sedimentation rate (ESR)
An elevated ESR is a non-specific sign of disease. It may be raised in renal failure, connective tissue disease and in acute or chronic infections.

Sodium
Hyponatraemia may be caused by:
- Diuretic therapy;
- Heart failure;
- Syndrome of inappropriate antidiuretic hormone (SIADH) secretion;

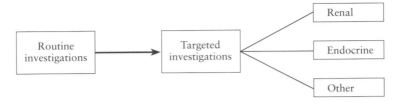

Figure 3.1 Sequence of investigations for hypertension.

Table 3.1 Routine initial investigations for all patients with confirmed hypertension.

Full blood count
ESR
Biochemistry
   Sodium, potassium
   Urea, creatinine
   Calcium, phosphate
   Fasting lipids (total cholesterol, triglycerides, LDL and HDL-cholesterol)
   Fasting glucose
   [Urate]*

Urine 'dipstick' analysis for microalbuminuria, proteinuria, microhaematuria
ECG
Chest X-ray

*Although serum urate is likely to be elevated in patients with hypertension, diabetes, dyslipidaemia or heart failure, it is a poor predictor of individual risk of coronary heart disease or stroke. It can, however, be measured if gout or urate nephrolithiasis are suspected.
ESR, erythrocyte sedimentation rate; HDL, high-density lipoprotein.

- The hyponatraemic hypertensive syndrome observed in severe renal artery stenosis.
    Hypernatraemia may occur in:
- Dehydration. Elderly patients are particularly susceptible to water loss. Resulting haemoconcentration may also manifest as increased haematocrit.
- Primary hyperaldosteronism (Conn's syndrome). Serum sodium concentrations are usually normal or low in hyperaldosteronism secondary to chronic renal failure.

Potassium
Hypokalaemia may occur in:
- Diuretic therapy. Both thiazide and loop diuretics cause hypokalaemia, which can precipitate arrhythmias in patients taking digoxin and in those who are otherwise predisposed to ventricular arrhythmias.
- Hyperaldosteronism (Conn's syndrome of hypertension, hypokalaemia, hypernatraemia, high plasma aldosterone and decreased plasma renin activity).
- Pseudoaldosteronism (hypertension, hypokalaemia, *low or undetect-*

able plasma aldosterone), as found in congenital adrenal hyperplasia, deoxycorticosterone-producing tumours, syndrome of apparent mineralocorticoid excess (AME), Liddle's syndrome and mineralocorticoid therapy.

• Renin-secreting tumour (children, very rare), which is usually benign and rarely malignant, is a cause of hypertension and hypokalaemia.

Hyperkalaemia may occur in:

• Renal failure;

• Therapy with angiotensin-converting enzyme (ACE) inhibitors in combination with potassium-sparing diuretics (spironolactone, amiloride).

Urea and creatinine
Despite the fact that the level of plasma creatinine is a poor indicator of glomerular filtration, it remains the most practicable measurement of renal function for screening purposes. Measurement of creatinine clearance or ethylenediamine tetra-acetic acid (EDTA) clearance should be reserved for hypertensive patients in whom secondary hypertension is suspected or in those with normal plasma creatinine and other signs of end-organ damage, such as left ventricular hypertrophy (LVH) or dysfunction.

Urate
Hyperuricaemia is found in association with hypertension, CHD and heart failure [1]. In addition, hyperuricaemia is associated with metabolic risk factors for CHD including hypertension [2,3], obesity [4,5], glucose intolerance [2–6], dyslipidaemia [7], hyperinsulinaemia and impaired glucose tolerance. The finding of hyperuricaemia should not be regarded as a cardiovascular risk factor, but as a pointer to other metabolic risk factors for CHD. In patients with heart failure, high serum uric acid levels are a marker of poor prognosis [8].

Calcium and phosphate
Hypercalcaemia may point towards primary hyperparathyroidism as a cause of hypertension.

Lipids
Dyslipidaemias, both familial and polygenic, act jointly with hypertension to promote atherosclerosis. All hypertensive patients should have measurement of total cholesterol, high-density lipoprotein (HDL)-cholesterol and triglycerides following an overnight fast. Lipid-lowering measures are an integral part of management of the hypertensive patient (Chapter 8).

Urinalysis
'Dipstick' testing for blood, glucose and protein should be performed in all hypertensive patients. Proteinuria and haematuria may point towards

hypertensive nephrosclerosis, glomerulonephritis, polycystic kidney disease, pyelonephritis and urogenital malignancies.

ECG

Although there is little justification for using the ECG as a screening test in asymptomatic individuals, its use in the screening of patients with hypertension is justified on the grounds that it can influence clinical management (e.g. prescribing aspirin or statins). All hypertensive patients have a resting 12-lead ECG, whether or not angina or MI is suspected. Up to 60% of elderly hypertensive patients have an abnormal ECG [9]. In the traditional literature on hypertension, particular emphasis has been placed on the use of the ECG to detect LVH. However, the most common cause of an abnormal ECG in hypertensive patients is not LVH, but CHD.

Coronary heart disease. The resting ECG is usually unhelpful in the diagnosis of angina [10], but it may be complementary if it shows evidence of a previous MI [11], which is likely to be found in ≈ 50% of cases [12,13]. Examples of ECG showing evidence of MI are shown in Fig. 3.2.

Significant ST segment depression may occur in up to 45% of hypertensive patients with a normal coronary angiogram. T-wave inversion is often disregarded and labelled as 'non-specific'. It should be noted, however, that such change may not be necessarily benign. The finding of ST depression, T-wave inversion, Q waves and left axis deviation increases the risk of future coronary events.

Left ventricular hypertrophy (LVH). Hypertension is the commonest cause of LVH in the general population. It should be noted, however, that an ECG pattern of LVH and/or 'strain' can also occur in other conditions which impose an increased resistance to LV outflow, such as aortic stenosis and mitral regurgitation. An LVH pattern may also be found in hypertrophic cardiomyopathy and dilated cardiomyopathy. Because of sustained, increased resistance to atrial inflow, the left atrium may also show hypertrophic changes.

The main electrical consequences of an increase in left ventricular mass are (Fig. 3.3):
• An increase in the amplitude of the waves 'crossing' the left ventricle — the R and S waves;
• A delay in the conduction of impulses through the LV wall.

Several sets of ECG diagnostic criteria have been proposed for the diagnosis of LVH (Table 3.2). It is noteworthy that limb lead criteria are more sensitive than chest lead criteria in obese individuals, whereas chest leads are more sensitive for lean individuals [14]. Although hypertensive LVH causes left axis deviation, it is important not to dismiss other causes, such as CHD, aortic stenosis and the fibrous degeneration of the anterior division of the left

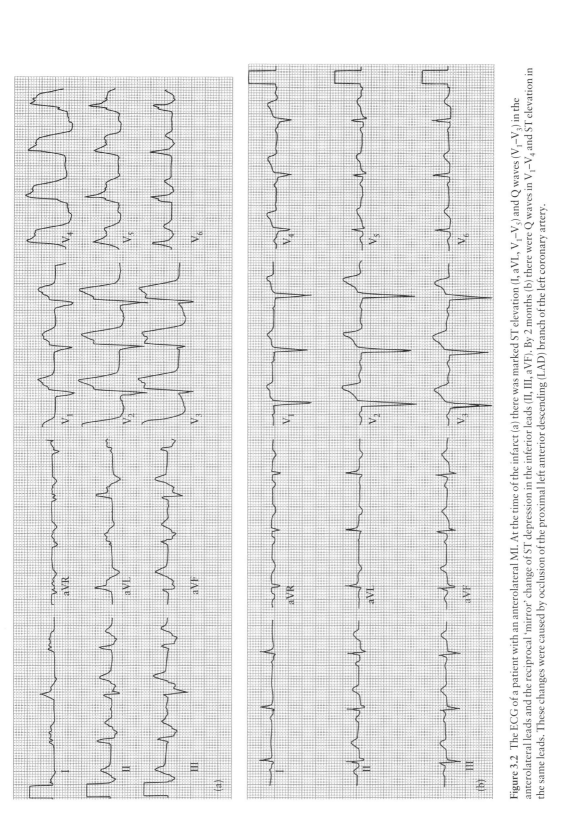

Figure 3.2 The ECG of a patient with an anterolateral MI. At the time of the infarct (a) there was marked ST elevation (I, aVL, V_1–V_5) and Q waves (V_1–V_3) in the anterolateral leads and the reciprocal 'mirror' change of ST depression in the inferior leads (II, III, aVF). By 2 months (b) there were Q waves in V_1–V_4 and ST elevation in the same leads. These changes were caused by occlusion of the proximal left anterior descending (LAD) branch of the left coronary artery.

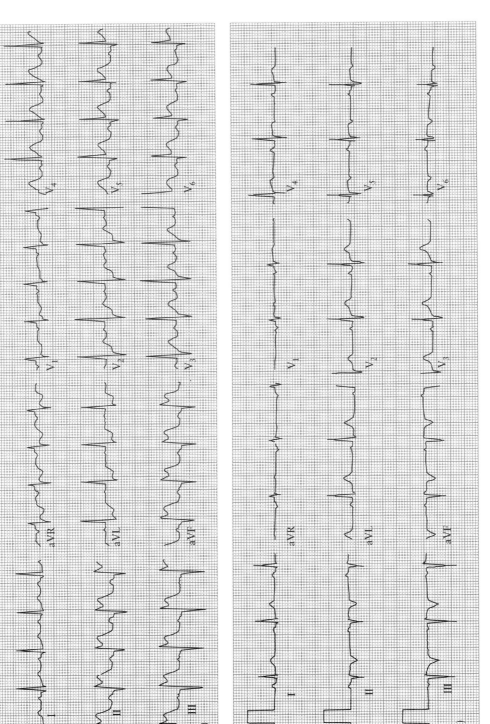

Figure 3.2 (*Cont'd*) ECG of a patient with an inferior MI. At the time of the infarct (c) there was marked ST elevation and Q waves in leads II, III and aVF, and leads V_5 and V_6. Reciprocal 'mirror' changes of ST depression are seen in the anterolateral leads (aVL, V_1, V_2). By 3 months (d) the ST segments return to baseline and Q waves are present in the inferior leads (II, III, aVF). T wave inversion is present in the inferior leads and leads V_5 and V_6. These changes were caused by occlusion of the right coronary artery.

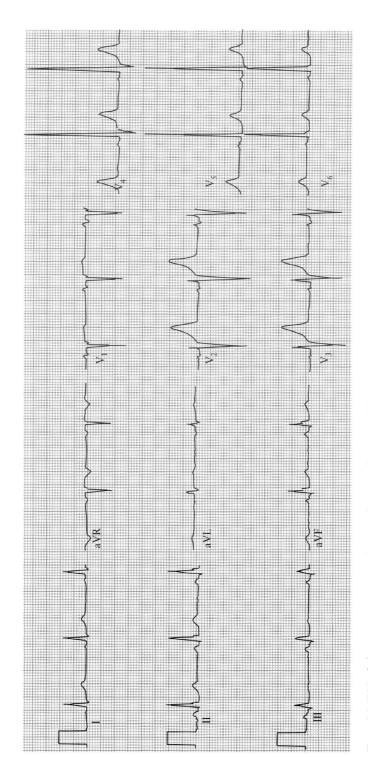

Figure 3.3 ECG of a hypertensive patient with LVH. This ECG of a 76-year-old hypertensive patient shows sinus rhythm and a normal QRS axis. The height of the R wave in leads V4 and V5 is > 35 mm, suggesting LVH.

Table 3.2 ECG criteria for left ventricular hypertrophy.*

Sokolow-Lyon voltage criteria
S wave in V_1 *plus* R wave in V_5 or V_6 > 35 mm

Sensitivity 22%
Specificity 100%

Cornell voltage criteria
R wave in aVL *plus* S wave in V_3 > 28 mm in men or > 20 mm in women

Sensitivity 42%
Specificity 96%

---

*From a validation study using autopsy findings (from [15] with permission of the American Heart Association).

bundle branch that occurs in the elderly. If the frontal QRS axis is deviated more than $-30°$, a left anterior hemiblock should be diagnosed.

Hypertrophy or ischaemia? Significant ST segment depression may occur in up to 45% of hypertensive patients with a normal coronary angiogram. Sometimes, therefore, it is often difficult to decide whether, in a hypertensive patient with chest pain, ST-segment depression and T-wave inversion should be taken as evidence of LVH or on-going myocardial ischaemia (Fig. 3.4). In such cases, the presence of chest pain at the time when the ECG was taken or ST segments and T-wave changes in subsequent ECGs would favour the diagnosis of ischaemia rather than LVH.

Left ventricular dysfunction. Although the ECG gives no indication of heart function, it is rarely normal in patients with heart failure. It is essential for the confirmation of sinus rhythm. The presence of Q-waves would suggest a MI. The presence of ECG signs of LVH together with a history of symptoms of heart failure would suggest hypertension as the cause in the absence of other apparent causes.

Chest X-ray. Prominence of the left ventricular border on the chest X-ray occurs in LVH but, in practice, the chest X-ray should not be used for the assessment of LVH. Although the relationship between heart size on the chest X-ray and left ventricular function is poor [16], the absence of radiological cardiomegaly should call into question a diagnosis of heart failure. The presence of radiological cardiomegaly represents an advanced stage of left ventricular dysfunction. The chest X-ray should be scrutinized for evidence of upper lobe venous dilatation, interstitial or alveolar oedema and pleural effusions (Fig. 3.5).

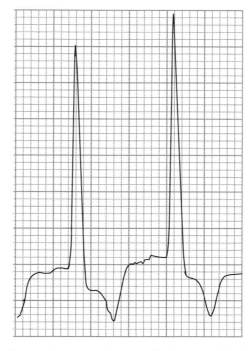

Figure 3.4 Hypertrophy or ischaemia? Both LVH and ischaemia and both together can produce ST-segment depression and T wave inversion.

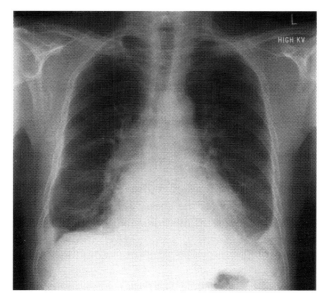

Figure 3.5 Chest X-ray of a patient with hypertensive heart failure. This chest X-ray from a 61-year-old hypertensive patient with heart failure shows an increase in size of the cardiac silhouette, prominence of the upper lobe veins, blunting of the costophrenic angles and increased shadowing in the lung parenchyma. This is consistent with cardiomegaly, upper lobe diversion of blood secondary to pulmonary venous hypertension, bilateral pleural effusions and oedema of the lung parenchyma.

TARGETED INVESTIGATIONS: FOCUSING ON END-ORGAN DAMAGE AND CO-EXISTENT CARDIOVASCULAR DISEASE

These should be considered in the following circumstances:
- If abnormalities emerge from the clinical history and examination, and routine investigations;
- In hypertension which responds poorly to drug therapy;
- If unexpected blood pressure elevations occur in hypertensive patients who are normally well controlled on drug therapy or in previously non-hypertensive individuals;
- In severe hypertension (≥ 180/110 mmHg) at presentation or during follow-up.

Before committing patients to extensive investigations, it is important to consider whether or not the results of the special investigations will influence clinical management. The investigations relating to causes of secondary hypertension are dealt with in Chapter 10. Other investigations which may be deemed appropriate in patients with essential hypertension are mainly geared towards determining the presence and degree of hypertensive end-organ damage and identifying coincidental disease.

Cardiovascular investigations

These are almost exclusively geared towards assessing hypertensive end-organ damage and concomitant heart disease.

Echocardiography. Echocardiography is more sensitive than electrocardiography or chest X-rays in detecting LVH [17–19]. Although echocardiographically detected LVH can predict mortality, it should be considered that no major outcome studies have addressed whether the use of echocardiographic information is of any value in the management of hypertension. For this and other reasons, most authorities [20,21] do not make firm recommendations on the general use of echocardiography for making decisions about management in patients who have mild hypertension but no clinical evidence of cardiac disease. If, however, the clinical assessment or routine investigations raise the possibility of cardiac disease, echocardiography may be very useful. It is more likely to be fruitful in the following categories:
- Patients in whom blood pressure is in the 'borderline' range for drug treatment, in whom the finding of LVH or asymptomatic left ventricular dysfunction will influence the decision to treat;
- Hypertensive patients with dyspnoea and/or reduced exercise tolerance, who may have left ventricular dysfunction;
- Patients with suspected valve disease, most commonly aortic valve disease;
- Patients with 'non-specific' changes on the ECG, such as T-wave inversion alone;
- Patients with angina and an abnormal ECG.

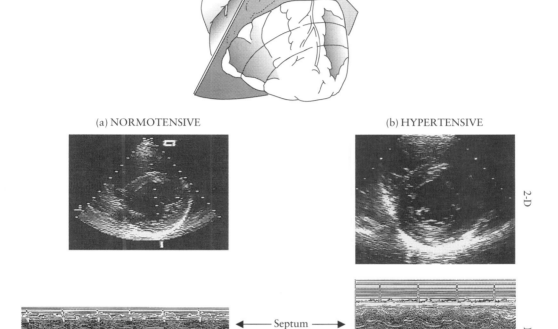

Figure 3.6 Echocardiography in the assessment of LVH. Two-dimensional and M-mode 'cut' of the left ventricle at a level just below the mitral valve in (a) a healthy individual, and (b) in a hypertensive patient with LVH. The scans show an increase in the thickness of the left ventricular septum and posterior ventricular walls.

M-mode [22] and two-dimensional echocardiography are simple and accurate tools for the determination of LVH and mass (Fig. 3.6) and left ventricular dysfunction (Fig. 3.7). As with most tests, echocardiography is of little value unless it is considered in the context of the whole clinical picture. An echocardiogram, comprising M-mode, two-dimensional views and Doppler flow measurements, can take up to 40 min to perform, involves

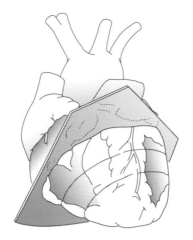

PLANE OF INTERROGATION

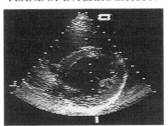

NORMAL LV FUNCTION   POOR LV FUNCTION

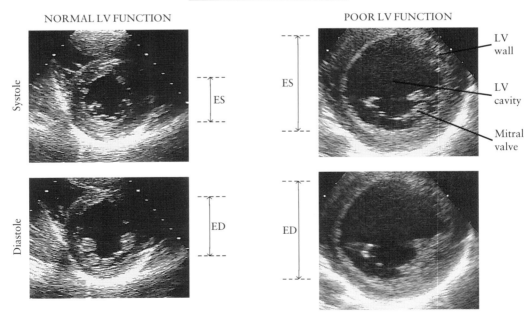

an experienced operator and expensive equipment. Furthermore, as with other tests, echocardiography is of little value unless it is considered in the context of the whole clinical picture and therefore, requires a cardiologist's opinion. Some centres have adopted a simplified echocardiographic procedure for the detection of LVH. This involves an M-mode echocardiogram on the long-axis view, at a level just below the mitral valve. This simple, albeit limited procedure, which takes 10 min to perform, may be considered by some clinics to be an appropriate screening test for patients with suspected LVH.

The notion that left ventricular ejection fraction (EF) is the best measure of cardiac function is an unfortunate myth. Limitations for the use of EF as a measure of heart function relates to the inherent limitations of the methodology used in calculations using M-mode and two-dimensional echocardiography (Fig. 3.7). It should also be noted that patients with clinically overt heart failure may have diastolic heart failure in the absence of systolic heart failure.

Doppler echocardiography is the investigation of choice in suspected aortic valve disease. It may reveal a forward gradient across the aortic valve in aortic stenosis and a regurgitant jet in aortic regurgitation.

Vascular ultrasonography. This investigation should be reserved for individuals with symptoms of cerebrovascular or peripheral vascular disease. The exception, however, is if an abdominal aortic aneurysm is found on examination. If an aneurysm is confirmed, a specialist vascular opinion should be sought.

Other investigations such as exercise testing, myocardial perfusion imaging and coronary angiography should be sought on the basis of clinical assessment and routine investigations. These are discussed in more detail in Chapter 5.

Renal investigations

Renal disease can be the cause or effect of hypertension. In fact, renal disease may be the trigger for hypertension and hypertension may then act

Figure 3.7 (*Opposite*) Echocardiography in the assessment of left ventricular function. Overall left ventricular systolic function is usually quantified in terms of the ejection fraction (EF), which is the fraction of the end-diastolic volume ejected from the left ventricle in systole. Echocardiography does not measure volume but rather, distances within a two-dimensional image. The standard method is to compute the EF using the left ventricular dimensions in end-systole (ES) and end-diastole (ED), which has considerable limitations. If, for example, the patient in question has previously had a MI affecting only the myocardial segment over which measurements are taken, the calculated overall left ventricular EF may be erroneously low. If, on the other hand, there has been an extensive MI sparing the segment over which measurements are taken, the calculated left ventricular EF may be erroneously high.

to promote further renal disease. There is, therefore, a fine line between the investigations aimed at identifying the cause and those aimed at identifying the effects of hypertension. The investigations relating to possible renal causes of secondary hypertension are dealt with in more detail on p. 144.

Glomerular filtration rate (GFR). Measurement of creatinine excretion over 24 h coupled with measurement of plasma creatinine provides a measure of creatinine clearance, which is calculated as follows:

$$\text{Creatinine clearance} = \frac{\text{urine creatinine (mmol l}^{-1}) \times \text{ml min}^{-1}}{\text{plasma creatinine (mmol l}^{-1})}$$

(Normal = 90–120 ml min^{-1}).

Proteinuria and microalbuminuria. In both insulin-dependent diabetes mellitus (IDDM) and non-insulin-dependent diabetes mellitus (NIDDM), proteinuria is associated with an increased risk of developing chronic renal failure. Microalbuminuria occurs early in the course of diabetes and has been shown to predict the development of nephropathy in patients with IDDM and, to a lesser extent, in patients with NIDDM [23]. They are defined as follows:
• Microalbuminuria: if two out of three 24-h urine collections over a period of 3 months yield an albumin excretion rate (AER) between 30 mg and 300 mg/24 h (20–200 µg min^{-1} or 300 mg l^{-1}).
• Macroalbuminuria: if two out of three 24-h urine collections yield an AER > 300 mg/24 h (> 200 µg min^{-1} or > 300 mg l^{-1}). In diabetic patients, this level indicates diabetic nephropathy.

Renal ultrasonography. This is more often useful in the investigation of a renal cause of secondary hypertension. The finding of small kidneys may point towards chronic hypertensive renal disease.

Intravenous urogram. The rapid-sequence intravenous urogram is currently preferred.

Isotope renography. This technique most commonly uses ^{99}Tc-DTPA (see Chapter 10). It is probably the most appropriate initial investigation in hypertensive patients who have been selected for investigation of renal artery stenosis on clinical grounds [24].

Renal arteriography. Conventional arteriography is the gold standard for investigation of renal artery stenosis [24], but it is currently being superseded by magnetic resonance angiography.

Renal biopsy. This can be performed if the above investigations do not help in deciding whether renal disease is the cause or effect of hypertension or if there is evidence of glomerular disease.

References

1 Leyva F, Anker SD, Swan J *et al.* Serum uric acid as an index of impaired oxidative metabolism in chronic heart failure. *Eur Heart J* 1997; 18: 858–865.
2 Beard JT. Serum uric acid and coronary heart disease. *Am Heart J* 1983; 106: 397–400.
3 Klein R, Klein BE, Omae T, Takeshita M, Hirota Y. The relationship of serum uric acid to hypertension and ischemic heart disease. *Arch Intern Med* 1973; 35: 173–178.
4 Bergman RN, Finegood DT, Ader M. Assessment of insulin sensitivity *in vivo*. *Endocrine Rev* 1985; 6: 45–86.
5 DeFronzo RA, Ferrannini E. The pathogenesis of non-insulin dependent diabetes: an update. *Medicine* 1982; 61: 125–140.
6 Modan M, Halkin H, Almog S *et al.* Hyperinsulinemia — a link between hypertension, obesity and glucose intolerance. *J Clin Invest* 1985; 75: 809–817.
7 Fox IH, John D, DeBruyne S, Dwosh I, Marliss EB. Hyperuricemia and hypertriglyceridemia: metabolic basis for the association. *Metabolism* 1985; 34: 741–746.
8 Anker SD, Leyva SD, Poole-Wilson PA, Coats AJS. Uric acid as an independent predictor of impaired prognosis in patients with chronic heart failure [abstract]. *J Am Coll Cardiol* 1998; 31: 154A.
9 SHEP Cooperative Research Group. Prevention of stroke by antihypertensive drug treatment in older persons with isolated systolic hypertension: final results of the Systolic Hypertension in the Elderly Program (SHEP). *JAMA* 1991; 265: 3255–3264.
10 Norrel M, Lythall D, Coghlan G *et al.* Limited value of the resting electrocardiogram in assessing patients with recent onset chest pain: lessons from a chest pain clinic. *Br Heart J* 1992; 67: 53–56.
11 Miranda CP, Lehmann KG, Froelicher VF. Correlation between resting ST-segment depression, exercise testing, coronary angiography, and long-term prognosis. *Am Heart J* 1991; 122: 1617–1628.
12 CASS. Principal Investigators and their associates. Coronary Artery Surgery Study (CASS): a randomized trial of coronary artery bypass surgery survival data. *Circulation* 1983; 68: 939–950.
13 Takato T, Hultgren HN, Detre C, Peduzzi P. The Veterans Administration cooperative study of stable angina: current status. *Circulation* 1982; 65 (Suppl. II): 60–67.
14 McLenachan JM, Henderson E, Morris KI, Dargie HJ. Electrocardiographic diagnosis of left ventricular hypertrophy: influence of body build. *Clin Sci* 1988; 75: 589–592.
15 Casale PN, Devereux RB, Alonso DR, Campo E, Kligfield P. Improved sex-specific criteria of left ventricular hypertrophy for clinical and computer interpretation of electrocardiograms: validation with autopsy findings. *Circulation* 1987; 75: 565–572.
16 McNamara RF, Carleen E, Moss AJ. Group and the Multicentre Post-infarction Research. Estimating left ventricular ejection fraction after myocardial infarction by various clinical parameters. *Am J Cardiol* 1988; 62: 192–196.
17 Romhilt DW, Bove KE, Nottis RJ *et al.* A critical appraisal of the electrocardiographic criteria for the diagnosis of left ventricular hypertrophy. *Circulation* 1969; 40: 185–195.

18   Devereau RB, Lutas EM, Casale PN *et al.* Standardization of M-mode echocardiographic left ventricular anatomic measurements. *J Am Coll Cardiol* 1984; 4: 1222–1230.

19   Woythaler JN, Singer SL, Kwan OL *et al.* Accuracy of echocardiography versus electrocardiography in detecting left ventricular hypertrophy: comparison with post-mortem mass measurements. *J Am Coll Cardiol* 1983; 2: 305–311.

20   Subcommittee to Develop Guidelines for the Clinical Application of Echocardiography. ACC/AHA guidelines for the clinical application of echocardiography. A report of the American College of Cardiology/American Heart Association Task Force on Assessment of Diagnostic and Therapeutic Cardiovascular Procedures. *J Am Coll Cardiol* 1990; 16: 1505–1528.

21   Haynes RB, Lacourcière Y, Rabkin SB *et al.* Diagnosis of hypertension in adults. *Can Med Assoc J* 1993; 149: 409–418.

22   Levy D, Garrison RJ, Savage DD *et al.* Prognostic implications of echocardiographically determined left ventricular mass in the Framingham Heart Study. *N Engl J Med* 1990; 322: 1561–1566.

23   Schmitz A, Veath M. Microalbuminuria: a major risk factor in non-insulin-dependent diabetes. A 10-year follow-up study of 503 patients. *Diabet Med* 1987; 5: 126–134.

24   Wilkinson R. Renal and renovascular hypertension. In: Swales J, ed. *Textbook of Hypertension*. Oxford: Blackwell Scientific Publications, 1994: 831–857.

4: Diagnostic and Treatment Thresholds, and Goals

Our views about hypertension are changing rapidly. Whereas in the past treatments were designed and applied on the basis of experimental and largely observational studies, there is now a fortunate tendency to rely on evidence derived from randomized clinical trials. The field of hypertension is not short of such studies. There is now little doubt that antihypertensive treatment reduces the risk of developing stroke and, to a lesser extent, coronary heart disease (CHD) (Fig. 4.1).

The recognition of the benefits from treating hypertension has paralleled the emergence of numerous working groups, task forces and committees dedicated to the management of hypertension. In the USA, the Joint National Committee (JNC) on Detection, Evaluation and Treatment of High Blood Pressure published its first recommendations in 1977, and these were followed by five further sets [2], the last one in 1997 [3]. Management guidelines have also been published from Canada [4], New Zealand [5], by the WHO/ISH joint conference [6] and the British Hypertension Society [7,8]. Such guidelines are largely in agreement, although there is still debate on details.

Whilst published guidelines are immensely helpful in managing hypertension, the clinician still faces the difficult choice as to which one to adopt. A problem is that the relatively unimportant discrepancies between them at times cloud the central messages upon which they all agree. The best practical compromise is to take recommendations from different sets of guidelines to suit individual clinical problems. Even then, there are issues that guidelines do not tackle, for example, how to manage hypertension in individuals with clinically occult atherosclerosis, be it CHD, cerebrovascular disease or peripheral vascular disease. In the following account, we shall draw on the latest recommendations published by international and national panels, with some modifications that we consider prudent in the light of other evidence.

CONFIRMING THE DIAGNOSIS

It is widely accepted that the diagnosis of mild-to-moderate hypertension should be made after repeated measurement over a period of time. In this respect, the following aspects are worth noting:

39

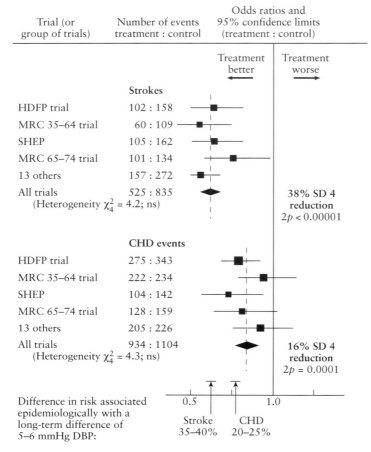

Figure 4.1 Benefits of antihypertensive treatment. Meta-analysis showing reduction in the odds of stroke and of coronary heart disease (CHD) in various trials of antihypertensive treatment. Solid squares represent the odds ratios (treatment/control) for the four larger trials and the properly stratified odds ratio for the combination of the 13 smaller trials. The size of the squares is proportional to the amount of information contributed by that study. Horizontal lines and diamonds denote 95% confidence intervals. Adapted with permission [1]. SD, standard deviation.

• Blood pressure, without intervention, can fall considerably over several months of observation [9].
• The diagnostic accuracy is improved by taking two [10] (but not more [11]) readings at one visit and taking the average reading.
• The number of visits at which blood pressure is assessed is more important than the number of measurements taken at any one visit [9,12].

Several authorities have proposed guidelines regarding the frequency and the period of assessment for patients with different levels of blood pressure. Such guidelines, however, do not cover all the possible combinations of blood pressure levels and clinical scenarios with which patients with elevated blood pressures might present to the clinician. Thus, in the absence of evidence from randomized trials, we recommend the following approach:

Systolic	Diastolic	Frequency of measurement
≥ 240	≥ 140	Consider hospital admission
200–240	120–140	Four occasions over 1 week
160–200	100–120	Four occasions over 1 month
140–160	90–100	Four occasions over 3 months
135–140	85–90	if plus other risks*: four occasions over 3 months if no other risks: yearly

*'Other risks' refers to the presence of 'target-organ damage', diabetes mellitus, cardiovascular disease or other cardiovascular risk factors.

Measurements in mmHg.

TREATMENT THRESHOLDS

Some authorities distinguish between the blood pressure thresholds at which hypertension should be diagnosed, the thresholds above which one should commence treatment and the threshold at which one should aim to maintain blood pressure during treatment. Whilst these questions are important from the research standpoint, this approach is not practical in current clinical management. We consider therefore that in the light of current knowledge, patients should be labelled as being hypertensive if, on clinical assessment, antihypertensive treatment is deemed necessary, taking into account the calculated risk of developing disease or dying. With reference to Professor Rose's principle, decisions on the threshold for both the diagnosis and treatment of hypertension should take into account whether medical intervention is going to 'do more good than harm'.

Age

Current guidelines on the diagnosis and management of hypertension apply to individuals ≥ 20 years of age. There is inadequate evidence as to the value of commencing antihypertensive treatment beyond the age of 79 years. On the basis of current evidence, treatment should not be withdrawn beyond 79 years of age in patients who are receiving treatment.

Risk stratification

In screening for hypertension, one should focus on those patients in whom hypertension will be most likely to incur mortality and morbidity and in

whom effective treatment is most likely to pay dividends (Table 4.1). Because more end-organ damage occurs if essential hypertension occurs in association with atherosclerosis, the clinician should focus on the following categories, in order of priority:
• Clinically overt *or occult* arteriosclerotic disorders, including CHD, cerebrovascular disease, renovascular disease, or peripheral vascular disease.
• Diabetes mellitus (both types I and II).
• Those who are at high risk of developing these diseases, i.e. those with cardiovascular risk factors.

Table 4.1 Effect of antihypertensive treatment on mortality in men with differing cardiovascular risk factor profiles*.

	65 years Non-smoker BP = 160/85 mmHg Normal ECG TC = 6.47 mmol l^{-1}	65 years Non-smoker BP = 160/95 mmHg Normal ECG TC = 6.47 mmol l^{-1}	74 years Smoker BP = 190/110 mmHg 'Ischaemic' ECG TC = 6.47 mmol l^{-1}
Stroke	83	71	22
Fatal or non-fatal MI	37	35	13
Other cardiovascular events	30	26	11

*Results are expressed as the number of men required to be treated with diuretic (hydrochlorothiazide 25 mg o.d. or 50 mg o.d.; amiloride 2.5 mg o.d. or 5 mg o.d.) to avoid one event in the three types of cardiovascular risk profiles. Adapted from the Medical Research Council trial of treatment of hypertension in older adults: Principal results [15].
BP, Blood pressure; TC, total cholesterol.

The principle of focusing on high risk groups is shared by all current management guidelines. Such guidelines, however, do not specify what measures to follow in patients with clinically occult cardiovascular disease. On the basis of current evidence, we advise that patients who are identified incidentally or opportunistically (history, examination or routine investigations) as having atheromatous cardiovascular disease, should be treated along the same lines as those who have clinically overt disease. Examples include patients with an 'old' MI on the screening ECG; and those who are found to have asymptomatic CHD on coronary angiography. A simplified version of the risk stratification system proposed by the 1999 WHO/ISH guidelines is shown in Fig. 4.2.

TREATMENT GOALS

The overall aim of treating hypertension is to reduce morbidity and mortality, which mainly occur as a result of cerebrovascular and CHD. Because these are also due to other factors, controlling blood pressure is only one of the goals of antihypertensive management. Formerly, opinions varied as to what fixed threshold should be aimed at during antihypertensive treatment. Much of this debate [8] related to the issue as to whether reductions below 125/85 mmHg lead to an increase in coronary events in patients with CHD [16]. In the recent HOT trial, comparison of clinical outcomes between the three blood pressure target groups of non-diabetic individuals (DBP ≤ 90, 85 or 80 mmHg) did not differ significantly. In diabetic patients, lowering diastolic blood pressure < 80 mmHg resulted in significant reductions in cardiovascular events [17]. Similarly, in the UKPDS 38, lowering blood pressure to 144/82 mmHg rather than to 154/87 mmHg was associated with significantly lower risks of major macrovascular events and microvascular disease outcomes [18]. Similar data are not available for patients with other associated conditions, such as CHD, heart failure, stroke, peripheral vascular disease, renal disease or retinopathy. However, in the light of the evidence available for diabetes, it would seem prudent to adopt similar blood pressure goals in patients with these conditions. Treatment goals are shown in Fig. 4.2.

Ambulatory blood pressure measurements

There is insufficient data at present to determine whether home measurements should be used in the diagnosis and management of hypertension. There is also considerable debate as to what levels of blood pressure measured using ambulatory blood pressure monitoring should be considered in the diagnosis of hypertension. Proposed thresholds for drug treatment of hypertension based on 24-hour ambulatory blood pressure measurements are as follows:

Diagnostic thresholds using ambulatory blood pressure monitoring		
	Normotensive	Definitely hypertensive
Daytime pressure	< 140/90	≥ 150/95
Night time pressure	< 120/75	≥ 130/80
24-h pressure	< 130/85	≥ 140/90

Suggested thresholds for 24-h ambulatory blood pressure for use in clinical practice. Levels have been rounded off for ease of use in clinical practice. Reproduced with permission from [13].

With regard to home measurement, the JNC advises that readings ≥ 135/85 mmHg should be considered elevated [14]. The following points, however, should be noted:

• There are no data on the use of self-measured blood pressure for initiating antihypertensive treatment.

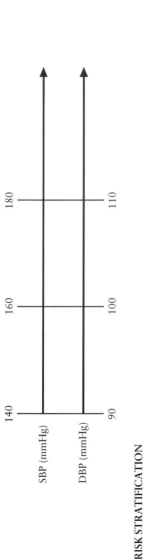

SBP (mmHg): 140 160 180

DBP (mmHg): 90 100 110

RISK STRATIFICATION

	LOW RISK	MEDIUM RISK	HIGH RISK
No risk factors, TOD or ACC	LOW RISK	MEDIUM RISK	HIGH RISK
Up to 2 risk factors	MEDIUM RISK	MEDIUM RISK	V HIGH RISK
≥ 3 risk factors ±TOD, ACC or diabetes or black race*	HIGH to V HIGH RISK	HIGH to V HIGH RISK	HIGH to V HIGH RISK

Risk of a major cardiovascular event occurring in the following 10 years: low, < 15%; medium, 15–20%; high, 20–30%; very high, ≥ 30%.

TREATMENT GOALS

ABSOLUTE RISK GROUP	BLOOD PRESSURE GOAL	LIPID GOAL	ASPIRIN
LOW RISK	Continue to monitor if: SBP > 140 ≤ 150 mmHg or DBP > 90 ≤ 95 mmHg Start drug treatment if SBP ≥ 150 mmHg or DBP ≥ 95 mmHg Aim for: **BP ≤ 140/90 mmHg** over 6 months	Continue to monitor total and LDL-cholesterol Aim for:	
MEDIUM RISK	Aim for: **BP ≤ 140/90 mmHg** over 6 months	Total cholesterol < 5.0 mmol l⁻¹ LDL–cholesterol < 3.0 mmol l⁻¹ with lifestyle advice and statins	Aspirin 75 mg o.d. for life to all treated, well controlled hypertensive patients
HIGH to V HIGH RISK	Aim for: **BP ≤ 130/85 mmHg** over 3 months	over 6 months	

Risk factors used for risk stratification are:
- Age: Men > 55 years, women > 65 years
- Smoking
- Total cholesterol > 6.5 mmol l⁻¹ (250 mg dl⁻¹)
- Family history of premature cardiovascular disease

Target Organ Damage includes:
- Left ventricular hypertrophy
- Proteinuria and/or elevation in plasma creatinine
- Ultrasound or radiological evidence of atherosclerosis
- Generalized or focal narrowing of the retinal arteries

Associated Clinical Conditions include:
- Cerebrovascular disease (ischaemic or haemorrhagic stroke or transient ischaemic attack)
- Heart disease (MI, angina, coronary revascularization, congestive heart failure)
- Renal disease (diabetic nephropathy, renal impairment)
- Vascular disease (including aortic aneurysm)
- Advanced hypertensive retinopathy (haemorrhages, exudates or papilloedema)

Figure 4.2 Diagnostic and treatment thresholds. The risk stratification table is largely based on that adopted by the WHO-ISH guidelines [19]. It has been simplified by amalgamating the group with '3 or more risk factors or TOD or diabetes' and the group with 'associated clinical conditions' into one group. Accordingly, the risk pertaining to this group is now quoted as high-to-very high. * On the basis that in African Americans, compared to the general population, hypertension develops at an earlier age, becomes more severe, and is associated with an 80% mortality from stroke, a 50% higher mortality from heart disease, and a 320% greater rate of target organ damage [20,21], black race has been added to the group with '3 or more risk factors or TOD, or ACC or diabetes'.

• There is scarce data on the distribution of self-monitored pressures in the normotensive and the hypertensive population.

• There have been no prospective studies addressing the relationship between self-measured blood pressure or its treatment and either morbidity or mortality.

References

1   Collins R, Peto R. Antihypertensive drug therapy: Effects on stroke and coronary heart disease. In: Swales JD, ed. *Textbook of Hypertension*. Oxford: Blackwell Scientific Publications, 1994: 1156–1164.

2   National High Blood Pressure Education Program, National Heart, Lung and Blood Institute. *The Fifth Report of the JNC on Detection, Evaluation and Treatment of High Blood Pressure*. National Institute of Health.

3   National Institutes of Health, National Heart, Lung and Blood Institute, National High Blood Pressure Education Program. *The Sixth Report of the Joint National Committee on the Prevention, Detection, Evaluation, and Treatment of High Blood Pressure*. National Institutes of Health, 1997.

4   Myers MG, Carruthers SG, Leenen FHH *et al*. Recommendations from the Canadian Hypertension Society Consensus Conference on the pharmacologic treatment of hypertension. *Can Med Assoc J* 1989; 140: 1141–1146.

5   Jackson R, Barhal P, Bills J *et al*. Management of raised blood pressure in New Zealand: a discussion document. *BMJ* 1993; 307: 107–110.

6   Zanchetti A, Chalmers J, Arakawa K *et al*. Summary of the 1993 WHO Society of Hypertension guidelines for the management of mild hypertension. *BMJ* 1993; 307: 1541–1546.

7   Swales JD, Ramsay LE, Coope JR *et al*. Treating mild hypertension. *BMJ* 1989; 298: 694–698.

8   Sever P, Beevers G, Bulpitt C, Lever A, Ramsay L, Reid J. Management guidelines in essential hypertension: report of the second working party of the British Hypertension Society. *BMJ* 1993; 306: 983–987.

9   Shepard DS. Reliability of blood pressure measurements: implications for designing and evaluating programs to control hypertension. *J Chronic Dis* 1981; 34: 191–209.

10 Donner A, Bull S. The mean versus the minimum as a criterion for hypertension screening. *J Chronic Dis* 1981; 34: 527–531.

11 Mathieu G, Biron P, Roberge F. 1: Blood pressure determinations during medical examinations: How many? *Can J Public Health* 1974; 65: 447–450.

12 Rosner B. Screening for hypertension some statistical observations. *J Chronic Dis* 1977; 30: 7–18.

13 O'Brien E. Ambulatory blood pressure measurement. In: O'Brien E, Beevers D, Marshall H, eds. *ABC of Hypertension*. London: BMJ Publishing Group, 1995: 28–34.

14 Tsuji I, Imai Y, Nagai K *et al*. Proposal of reference values for home blood pressure measurement: prognostic criteria based on a prospective observation of the general population in Ohasama. *Japan Am J Hypertens* 1997; 10: 409–418.

15 MRC Working Party. Medical Research Council Trial of treatment of hypertension in older adults: principal results. *BMJ* 1992; 304: 405–412.

16 Cruickshank JM, Thorpe JM, Zacharias FJ. Benefits and potential harm of lowering high blood pressure. *Lancet* 1987; i: 581–584.

17   Hansson L, Zanchetti A, Carruthers SG *et al.* for the HOT Study Group. Effects of intensive blood pressure lowering and low-dose aspirin in patients with hypertension: principal results of the Hypertension Optimal Treatment (HOT) randomised trial. *Lancet* 1998; 351: 1755–1762.

18   UK Prospective Diabetes Study Group. Efficacy of atenolol and captopril in reducing risk of macrovascular and microvascular complications in type 2 diabetes: UKPDS 39. *BMJ* 1998; 317: 713–720.

19   WHO. 1999 World Health Organisation-International Society of Hypertension guidelines for the management of hypertension. *J Hypertens* 1999; 17: 151–183.

20   Singh GK, Kochanek KD, MacDorman MF. Advance report of final mortality statistics, 1994. *Mon Vital Stat Rep* 1996; 45: 1–76.

21   Klag MJ, Whelton PK, Randall BL *et al.* End-stage renal disease in African-American and white men: 16-year MRFIT findings. *JAMA* 1997; 277: 1293–1298.

Part 2 Hypertension in Context

5: Cardiac Disease

Hypertension is, and should be regarded by the clinician, as a cardiovascular risk factor. Because stroke and heart disease are the most important contributors to morbidity and mortality in hypertensive patients, management of hypertension must be geared towards reducing the overall risk of developing these conditions. Overall management of the hypertensive patient will also entail specific management of coronary heart disease (CHD), heart failure, cardiac arrhythmias and valvular disease. Management of these conditions will not only focus on treating symptoms but also on improving life expectancy. Most of the drugs used for these purposes are also used in the management of hypertension.

Traditionally, the literature on hypertension has focused more on left ventricular hypertrophy (LVH) than on CHD. In fact, hypertension is more commonly associated with CHD, in the form of angina or myocardial infarction (MI), than with LVH. Because the presence of CHD will influence antihypertensive management to a greater extent than the presence of LVH, emphasis should be placed on its early diagnosis and treatment. This chapter deals with aspects of cardiac disease that are likely to be encountered in the management of hypertensive patients.

THE VASCULATURE: MYOCARDIAL INFARCTION AND ANGINA

Myocardial infarction has a devastating effect on health, at both individual and population levels. Following an MI, a quarter of patients die before reaching hospital. About 10% of those who reach hospital die in the first year post-MI and the subsequent annual death rate is 5%.

Hypertension is a major risk factor for MI [1]. In the Framingham study, in up to 60% of cases of untreated hypertension, death resulted from MI or heart failure [2]. The risk of coronary death increases progressively with increasing blood pressure, as shown by the Multiple Risk Factor Intervention Trial (MRFIT, 316 099 subjects, 11.6 years' follow-up) [3]. Following an MI, isolated systolic hypertension [4] and combined systolic and diastolic hypertension [5,6] are major determinants of a worse prognosis, particularly in the case of anterior MI [7].

The mechanistic link between hypertension and CHD remains uncertain. Hypertension may cause vascular disease by promoting endothelial damage [8], by increasing transport of lipoproteins into vessel walls and by reducing oxygen delivery to the arterial intima. Whether these factors are the cause of vascular disease or a manifestation of a denominator common to both hypertension and CHD is a matter of active debate.

Diagnosis

Points to note in the history of angina include its precipitants, such as exertion, food intake and cold weather. One should consider the atypical presentations of MI [9] (Table 5.1) and the fact that silent MIs are common in middle-aged males [10], particularly in the context of diabetes and hypertension [11]. In the Framingham study, between 20 and 60% of non-fatal MIs unrecognized by the patient were discovered on subsequent ECGs [11,12] or autopsies.

Patients with angina are likely to have had an MI (Table 5.2) and may already have significant reductions in left ventricular function (Table 5.3). The clinical examination may be uninformative, but in those with a previous MI, there may be cardiomegaly or signs of heart failure.

Table 5.1 Atypical presentations of myocardial infarction.

Heart failure — *de novo* or acute-on-chronic
Classical angina pectoris, without a prolonged attack
Atypical location of chest pain
Stroke
Syncope
Acute indigestion
Peripheral embolism
Overwhelming weakness
Apprehension or nervousness
Sudden mania or psychosis

Reproduced with permission from Bean, W.B. Masquerade of myocardial infarction. *Lancet* 1977; 1: 1044. © The Lancet Ltd. [9].

Table 5.2 History of myocardial infarction in patients with angina.

Study	%
CASS	59
ECSSG	45
VA study	60

Percentage of patients with previous myocardial infarction in the Coronary Artery Surgery Study (CASS, 467/780 patients); the European Coronary Surgery Study (ECSSG, 349/768 patients); and the Veterans Administration (VA) study (411/686).

Table 5.3 Prevalence of left ventricular dysfunction in 2520 patients referred for coronary artery bypass surgery.

	%
Normal LV function	55.5
Mild reduction	27.8
Moderate reduction	14.7
Severe reduction	2.0
Previous MI	51.8

Reproduced from [12] with permission of Oxford University Press, UK.

Angina is not a diagnosis, insofar as it gives no indication of its cause. In this sense, it is as uninformative as the diagnosis of anaemia; angina could be a result of stenosis in a small distal branch of a coronary artery, in which case it is unlikely to have a fatal outcome, or of stenosis of the main stem of the left coronary artery, which is likely to have fatal consequences. It should be noted that neither the severity nor localization of pain give any indication of the arterial territory involved. On the other hand, hypertensive patients with angina may not necessarily show stenosing epicardial CHD on coronary angiography [13], even though there may be evidence of myocardial ischaemia on myocardial perfusion scanning [14]. There is uncertainty as to whether microvascular disease is the culprit of angina in some hypertensive patients.

Investigations
All patients with angina should undergo a number of routine investigations, most of which are readily available to the general practitioner. Targeted investigations should proceed if abnormalities arise on these routine investigations (Table 5.4).

ECG. Up to 75% of patients with angina have a normal resting 12-lead ECG when first seen. Angina, however, is more likely if the ECG is abnormal and in particular, if it shows evidence of an 'old' MI. It should be noted that as well as being associated with LVH, hypertension is also associated with left atrial hypertrophy and atrial fibrillation (p. 75). Examples of ECGs showing MI are shown on pp. 27–29. Briefly, the steps to follow for the ECG diagnosis of MI are:

1 *Identify abnormalities of the QRS complex*:
   • q waves which either are ≥ 0.04 s in duration (excluding aVR and III) *or* that have a depth which is more than a quarter of the ensuing R wave (excluding aVR and III) are considered pathological Q waves;
   • QS complexes (excluding aVR and III);

Table 5.4 Assessment of patients with angina.

History and examination

Routine investigations
Full blood count
U+Es, creatinine
Fasting glucose
Lipids (cholesterol, HDL-C, LDL-C, triglycerides)
Creatine kinase / Troponin T*
Chest X-ray
ECG

Targeted investigations†
Exercise test
Stress [201]Thallium imaging
Echocardiogram if ECG abnormal
Coronary angiography

---

*If MI is thought to have occurred within 3 days.
†Suggest referral to cardiologist.
HDL-C, high-density lipoprotein cholesterol, LDL-C, low-density lipoprotein cholesterol.

- R waves absent or with inappropriately low voltage ('poor R-wave progression').

2 *Identify the 'transmural' extent of the infarction:*
- Transmural: there will be total loss of R waves in the leads overlying the infarct;
- Part of left ventricular thickness: the amplitude of the residual R waves overlying the infarct is diminished.

3 *Identify the distribution of the QRS abnormalities:*

Anterior	*Anteroseptal*	*Anterolateral*	*Inferior*	*Posterior*
Some of the group V_1–V_3 plus some of the group V_4–V_6	V_1, V_2, V_3	V_4, V_5, V_6 aVL and II	II, III, aVF	V_1, V_2 ('mirror' changes)

The above features can also occur in any condition that causes myocardial necrosis, including myocarditis.

Exercise testing. An exercise test (Fig. 5.1) should be considered in all patients with stable angina. As a diagnostic tool, the exercise test has a specificity of 88–97% and a sensitivity of 54–80% [15–17], with the lowest figures in women. Apart from being useful in diagnosis, exercise testing is also valuable in prognostic stratification; the greater the ST depression observed, the greater is the chance of subsequent coronary events. If the test is requested for diagnostic purposes, all anti-anginal treatment must be stopped

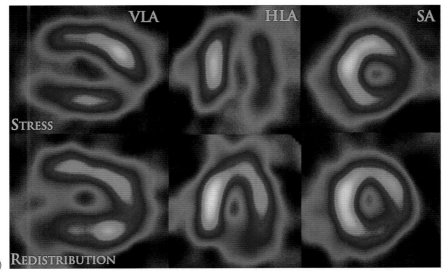

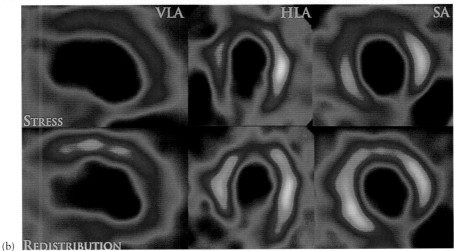

Plate 5.1 Stress thallium-201 (^{201}Tl) imaging in coronary heart disease. In ^{201}Tl imaging, defects in the myocardial thallium distribution will occur in non-viable areas (e.g. infarct) and in viable regions with reduced blood flow (e.g. an ischaemic zone distal to a haemodynamically significant coronary artery stenosis) when a 'stressing' agent such as dobutamine is administered. (a) This shows reversible ischaemia of the lateral wall and apex in a patient with a tight stenosis of the circumflex artery (a branch of the left coronary artery). The ischaemia is best seen in the horizontal (HLA) and short axis (SA) views with just the apical component visible in the vertical long axis (VLA). There is no evidence of significant myocardial damage after redistribution. (b) This shows a diffuse abnormality throughout the anterior wall, apex, inferior wall and septum in the enlarged heart of a patient with heart failure from hypertension. The redistribution study shows improvement in most areas, but this is least marked in the inferior wall and apex. There is no further significant improvement after re-injection, indicating that there is partial thickness infarction of the inferior wall and apex. There has been considerable remodelling of the heart. (Illustrations kindly provided by Dr Dudley Pennell.)

[facing page 54]

Table 5.5 Indications and contra-indications to exercise testing.

Indications
As a complementary diagnostic test of myocardial ischaemia
Evaluation of disease severity and response to anti-anginal therapy
Evaluation of exercise-induced arrhythmias

Absolute contra-indications
Acute MI
Recent unstable angina
Known left main stem disease
Severe aortic stenosis
Any generalized systemic illness, including myopericarditis
Physical incapacity, such as in the elderly, the obese and those with musculoskeletal disorders or
    intermittent claudication
Uncontrolled hypertension–dangerous and may yield false-positive results

Relative contra-indications
Absence of a history of chest pain–the number of falsely positive results [16, 17] are likely to
    mislead clinical management
Left bundle branch block–invalidates ST segment analysis
ST-segment depression at rest in patients with angina
Hypertrophic obstructive cardiomyopathy (HOCM)

---

on the morning of the test. If, however, the test is required for assessment of the response to anti-anginal treatment, the usual medication should be continued. Because of the considerable expertise needed to interpret the findings of an exercise test, all patients in whom exercise testing is contemplated should be referred to a cardiologist. The indications and contra-indications for exercise testing are shown in Table 5.5.

Myocardial perfusion imaging. This should be reserved for patients who are unable to perform an exercise test or those whose abnormalities on the resting ECG, such as left bundle branch block, preclude interpretation of the exercise ECG. The principle of this technique relies on the selective uptake of the radioisotope [201]Thallium by perfused areas of myocardium: unperfused myocardium, such as in infarctions, shows up as absent thallium intake, whereas regions of reduced perfusion show up as differences in regional uptake (Plate 5.1, facing p. 54). The technique can be used in conjunction with measures that 'stress' the myocardium, such as exercise or the intravenous administration of adenosine, dipyridamole, dobutamine or arbutamine.

Stress echocardiography. This is an alternative to thallium scanning. It consists of identifying areas of the myocardium with impaired contractility in response to exercise or pharmacological 'stress', usually dobutamine. The technique requires considerable expertise.

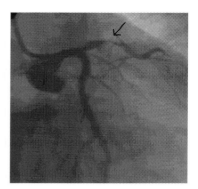

Figure 5.2 Coronary angiogram in coronary heart disease. Arrow points to a critical stenosis of the left anterior descending (LAD) branch of the left coronary artery.

Coronary angiography. This remains the gold standard for the diagnosis of coronary heart disease (Fig. 5.2). Generally, the procedure should be considered with a view to revascularization.

Symptomatic treatment of angina

On the basis of current evidence [18], we recommend the following drugs for the symptomatic treatment of patients with angina, whether or not they are hypertensive:

β-Blockers. The $β_1$-selective agents, such as atenolol 25–50 mg o.d., metoprolol 25–100 mg b.d. and bisoprolol 5–20 mg o.d. are the first choice drugs for patients with angina. It has been shown that patients taking β-blockers for hypertension are less likely to suffer a vascular event. Patients taking β-blockers who have had an MI have a lower mortality [19,20]. Patients should be warned not to stop β-blockers suddenly, or allow them to run out, as this may precipitate a coronary event [21].

Calcium antagonists. If β-blockers are not tolerated or if symptoms are not controlled, long-acting dihydropyridines, such as amlodipine 2.5–10 mg o.d., should be considered. Short-acting dihydropyridines should be avoided in patients with angina or with hypertension, given the current concerns that these agents may increase mortality. The negative chronotropic properties of verapamil and, to a lesser extent, diltiazem, may preclude the addition of a β-blocker. They are, however, very effective antianginal agents.

Nitrates. Glyceryl trinitrate (GTN) should be prescribed on an 'as required' basis to all patients with angina. Long-acting preparations of isosorbide mononitrate should be considered in those who do not tolerate β-blockers or long-acting dihydropyridines or those in whom symptoms are not controlled on these agents. Addition of isosorbide dinitrate or nitrate patches to β-blockers produces no additional benefit, whereas addition of isosorbide monotritrate is effective. Only those preparations which provide a 'nitrate-free' period and which therefore avoid nitrate tolerance should be considered.

Potassium channel openers. Nicorandil should be considered as second-line and as an alternative in patients who cannot tolerate a β-blocker (asthma, obstructive airways disease).

It is unclear whether, in the management of angina, addition of a third anti-anginal drug provides additional benefit [22–24].

Drug treatment of angina

Symptom control
β-blockers*
Calcium antagonists
Nitrates
Potassium channel openers

Prevention of MI
Aspirin*
Statins*
β-blockers*

*These drugs have been shown to reduce morbidity and mortality in randomized controlled trials.

Secondary prevention of myocardial infarction

The consequences of an MI are catastrophic (Table 5.6). There is now indisputable evidence that aspirin, β-blockers, ACE inhibitors and statins reduce mortality and morbidity following an MI (Table 5.7) [25]. Antihypertensive

Table 5.6 Consequences of a myocardial infarction within 6 years*.

	Men	Women
Sudden death	13	6
Further MI	23	31
Angina	41	34
Heart failure	20	20
Stroke	9	18

*Percentage of individuals succumbing to the above conditions following a myocardial infarction.

Table 5.7 Benefits of secondary prevention per 1000 patient years of treatment.

Aspirin	16 deaths/MIs/strokes
β-blocker	13 deaths, 5 MIs
ACE inhibitor	
MI complicated by LVF	45 deaths
LV dysfunction post-MI	12 deaths, 9 MIs, 16 cases of CHF
Statin	6 deaths, 12 MIs, 11 CABG or PTCA
Smoking cessation	27 deaths
Total	119 deaths including smoking cessation
	92 deaths excluding smoking cessation

Adapted with permission from [25].

management is an integral part of secondary prevention of MI, and should run hand in hand with other specific therapies.

Drugs used in the secondary prevention of MI*

Aspirin*
β-blockers*
ACE inhibitors*
Statins*
Oestrogen-replacement therapy

*These drugs have been shown to reduce morbidity and mortality in randomized controlled trials.

Non-pharmacological measures. These have been dealt with in Chapter 11 and are summarized in Table 5.8.

Pharmacological treatment

Aspirin. In individuals with CHD, aspirin reduces the risk of subsequent non-fatal ischaemic strokes, non-fatal MI, and total cardiovascular mortality in patients with unstable or stable angina, previous MI, previous transient ischaemic attacks or ischaemic stroke, following coronary artery bypass graft surgery and thrombolysis [26–34], and in acute evolving MI [29]. Benefits in survivors of an MI include a 12% reduction in death, a 31% reduction in reinfarction, and a 42% reduction in non-fatal stroke [34]. The benefit of aspirin in secondary prevention extends to women, the elderly, hypertensives and diabetics [33,35,36].

Unless there is a definite history of hypersensitivity (aspirin-induced bronchoconstriction, angio-oedema, urticaria, rhinitis) or a high risk of bleeding

Table 5.8 Lifestyle modifications for hypertensive patients with coronary heart disease.*

- Stop smoking
- Lose weight to keep BMI between 20 and 25 kg m^{-2}. Aim to lose 0.5–1 kg week^{-1} (not more) by avoiding fatty foods, sugar and alcohol. Crash diets do not help in the long term
- Limit alcohol intake to 28 units per week in men and to 21 units per week in women, without bingeing
- Walk briskly for ~45 min per day on most days of the week
- Keep a good diet for reducing coronary risk:
  Avoid processed foods
  Keep daily salt (sodium chloride) intake < 6 g day^{-1} by†:
    Avoiding processed foods and other salty foods
    Avoiding adding salt at the table
  Keep a low daily total and saturated fat intake
  Eat fresh fruit and vegetables with every meal
  Eat foods containing soluble fibre at least once a day
  Eat fish at least three times a week

*Advice on all points mentioned is supported by data from observational studies rather than randomized prospective studies.
†Whether salt intake should be reduced in normotensive patients is a contentious issue which has not been adequately addressed by any study.
BMI, body mass index.

(*active* peptic ulceration and *not* just a history of ulcers, recent injury or bleeding diathesis), life-long aspirin prophylaxis is recommended for all patients with atherosclerosis, such as those with angina, confirmed MI, as well as those with previous stroke, transient ischaemic attack, coronary or peripheral artery bypass surgery or angioplasty.

> A dose of 300 mg should be given immediately to all patients in whom MI is suspected, before transfer to hospital. If the diagnosis is confirmed, the dose should be switched to 75 mg o.d. on the second day of hospital admission and continued indefinitely.

In addition, aspirin should be given to all patients with asymptomatic atherosclerosis (as evidenced on peripheral, coronary or cerebral angiography or ultrasound examination) and to all treated hyperactive patients whose blood pressure is well controlled.

There are no clinical outcome data on other antiplatelet agents such as sulphinpyrazone and dipyridamole and therefore, these agents are not currently recommended in the primary or secondary prevention of CHD.

β-Blockers. β-blockers have been shown to produce a 20% reduction in long-term mortality and a 34% reduction in sudden cardiac death in survivors of MI [37–43]. They also reduce the incidence of MI in non-diabetic, hypertensive men and women [44]. The greatest reductions are seen in patients who have suffered an extensive anterior MI, those with compensated heart failure, asymptomatic left ventricular dysfunction or cardiac dysrhythmias. For this reason, β-blockers are the ideal antihypertensive agent for hypertensive patients who have had an MI.

> All survivors of Q-wave or non-Q-wave MI [45], hypertensive or normotensive, should be on life-long treatment with a β-blocker, unless contra-indicated. Treatment should ideally be started within 24 h of an MI.

Statins. The benefits of secondary prevention of treatment with 'statins' (inhibitors of 3-hydroxy-3-methylglutaryl coenzyme A (HMG-CoA) reductase) are undoubted. The effects of simvastatin and pravastatin on plasma cholesterol and cardiovascular events are shown in Table 5.9. Reductions in cardiovascular events and mortality in the 4S [46], CARE [47] and LIPID [48] trials were achieved in patients with only modest elevations in plasma cholesterol levels (4S: 5.5–8.0 mmol l⁻¹; CARE: < 6.2 mmol l⁻¹; LIPID: 4.0–7.0 mmol l⁻¹). A pooled analysis of coronary angiographic and carotid ultrasound studies with pravastatin revealed that a reduction of 52% in major coronary events paralleled a reduction in low-density lipoprotein (LDL)-cholesterol of 28% ($P = 0.006$) [49]. These studies pose a considerable challenge to those who are reluctant to use statins in patients with CHD. The subject is dealt with in detail in Chapter 8.

Oestrogen-replacement therapy. There is limited, albeit impressive, data from observational studies to support the use of oestrogen supplementation in postmenopausal women with CHD. However, the HERS study, the only randomized, controlled study of oestrogen therapy in postmenopausal women with CHD, has cast a shadow over its use in secondary prevention (Chapter 9).

Anti-arrhythmic therapy. Trials of anti-arrhythmic therapy aimed at suppressing ventricular ectopy in survivors of MI have shown an excess mortality compared to placebo (CAST study). D-Sotalol has proved disappointing (SWORD study). In contrast, two recent trials suggest that amiodarone may decrease ventricular fibrillation and death from arrhythmia, although no effect on total mortality emerged (CAMIAT, EMIAT). Thus, β-blockers are the only anti-arrhythmic drugs that have confidently been shown to improve prognosis in MI survivors. Trials on the prognostic value of implantable defibrillators in high risk patients are awaited.

Table 5.9 Trials of statins in the secondary prevention of MI.

Study	Subjects	Age of subjects (years)	Duration (years)	Situation	Drug used	Baseline TC (mmol l⁻¹)	Reduction in TC (%)	Reduction in LDL-C (%)	Significant outcomes*
4S [46]	3617 men 827 women	35–40	4.9–6.3	Secondary prevention	Simvastatin 20–40 mg o.d.	5.5–8.0	25	35	↓ Overall mortality by 30% ↓ CHD deaths by 42% ↓ Coronary events by 34%
CARE [47]	3583 men 576 women	21–75	4.0–6.2	Secondary prevention	Pravastatin 40 mg o.d.	<6.2	20	28	↓ Coronary events by 24% ↓ Revascularization events by 27%
LIPID† [48]	7498 men 1516 women	31–75	6.1	Secondary prevention	Pravastatin 40 mg o.d.	4.0–7.0	18	25	↓ Overall mortality by 22% ↓ Revascularization events by 20% ↓ Fatal and non-fatal MI by 24%

*p at least < 0.05 in all outcomes shown.
†The LIPID study also recruited patients with a history of unstable angina.

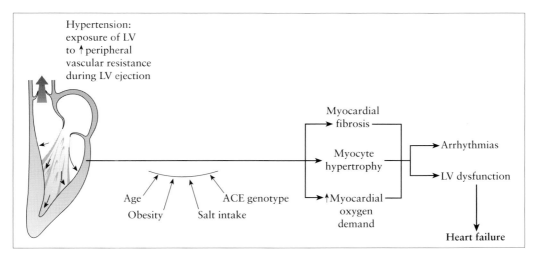

Figure 5.3 Pathophysiology of left ventricular hypertrophy. In hypertension, aortic valve opening during early left ventricular (LV) ejection exposes the LV to high pressures. With prolonged exposure to elevated pressures, the left ventricular wall thickens as a result of myocyte hypertrophy. Compensatory mechanisms ultimately become maladaptive when the LV approaches a critical mass [63], after which appreciable impairments in LV distensibility, relaxation and compliance occur. With increasing LVH there is increased myocardial oxygen demand and reduced myocardial coronary reserve. These factors, together with micronecrosis and fibrosis resulting from microvascular disease, add to myocardial dysfunction. The development of LVH is not only influenced by the magnitude and duration of the blood pressure load, but also by gender, age, catecholamines, angiotensin II, insulin, sodium balance, adiposity, heart rate and contractility, and variations in the ACE and angiotensinogen receptor (AT_1) gene. These factors act jointly to 'remodel' the left ventricle. Late in the development of hypertensive heart disease, the process of remodelling leads to LV dilatation and an impairment of overall LV function. The appearance of radiological or clinical signs of cardiac failure indicates a late stage of hypertensive heart disease.

THE MYOCARDIUM: LEFT VENTRICULAR HYPERTROPHY

Left ventricular hypertrophy (LVH) (Fig. 5.3) is end-organ damage and not surprisingly, it emerges as a potent 'risk factor' for CHD and heart failure in cohort and population studies, independent of clinic blood pressure levels, cigarette smoking and hypercholesterolaemia [50–53]. In the Framingham study, the presence of ST segment and T wave repolarization abnormalities ('left ventricular strain pattern') was associated with a sixfold increase in cardiac deaths over a follow-up period of 20 years [54]. Furthermore, the mortality in patients with angiographically proven CHD or following an acute MI doubles in the presence of LVH [55,56]. LVH carries a mortality similar to non-occlusive, triple vessel CHD [57]. There is evidence suggesting that this risk is attributable to complex ventricular tachyarrhythmias [58].

It is well established that antihypertensive treatment reduces LVH and that this occurs in proportion to its blood-pressure lowering effects [59–61]. Moreover, there is some evidence to suggest that regression of LVH achieved with antihypertensive treatment leads to reductions in cardiovascular events [62]. Nevertheless, prospective clinical outcome data on the effects of treating LVH *per se* is lacking. Some drugs, such as ACE inhibitors, appear to have a specific effect on LVH which is independent of blood-pressure lowering effects. This, however, has not been adequately explored in clinical trials.

Treatment

No controlled comparative trials of sufficient size and duration have explored which drug classes are the most effective at reducing cardiovascular events in hypertensive LVH. In recent meta-analyses [59,60], ACE inhibitors appear to be superior to calcium antagonists, thiazide diuretics and β-blockers at reducing LVH. It must be noted, however, that meta-analyses are inherently limited, insofar as they involve varying patient selection criteria and variations in the methods used to measure LVH. Nevertheless, the recent RACE study of 193 patients has demonstrated that for the same reduction in blood pressure, left ventricular mass was reduced by ramipril, but not by atenolol [64]. Further prospective randomized, comparative trials are clearly needed; but in the meantime, we recommend that ACE inhibitors be considered in patients with LVH. Their metabolic neutrality and their unsurmounted beneficial effects in patients with left ventricular dysfunction should also influence this decision.

HEART FAILURE AND LEFT VENTRICULAR DYSFUNCTION

The average prognosis of heart failure is similar to that of some cancers (Table 5.10). Hypertension is the most common antecedent of heart failure in the general population [2,65,66]. In the Framingham study, hypertension alone or in combination with CHD, accounted for ≈ 70% of cases of heart failure (Fig. 5.4) [67]. The pathophysiology of left ventricular function resulting from MI is illustrated in Fig. 5.5. As shown in Fig. 5.6, once left ventricular dysfunction develops in a patient with CHD, it becomes the single most important prognostic factor. As well as CHD, patients with hypertensive

Table 5.10 Five-year survival in heart failure and cancer.

Chronic heart failure	38%
Lung cancer (small cell, T_2N_1)	20–45%
Colorectal cancer (Dukes' C_1)	30–40%

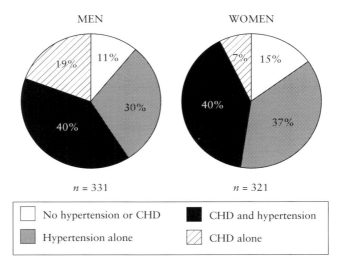

Figure 5.4 Prevalence of coronary heart disease (CHD) and hypertension (HT) alone or in combination in patients with heart failure. Adapted from the Framingham Heart Study [68]. Reproduced with permission from Poole-Wilson, P.A. *et al. Heart Failure* 1997, p. 281. Churchill Livingstone.

heart failure frequently have other conditions (Table 5.11) and each of these should be specifically addressed. It is often tempting to label a patient as having heart failure and overlook the underlying cause.

Diagnosis

Symptoms. These include breathlessness, ankle swelling, a reduction in exercise capacity and fatigue.

Signs. These include pitting gravitational oedema, a raised jugular venous pressure, hepatojugular reflux and hepatomegaly, all of which result from systemic venous congestion [70]. Peripheral oedema may be absent in adequately treated patients, or even in the presence of severe left ventricular dysfunction. Tachycardia and a raised jugular venous pressure are inconsistent findings, even in patients with confirmed heart failure [71]. The apex beat is not always an accurate measure of cardiomegaly. A third heart sound and pulmonary crepitations are not specific to heart failure and lend themselves to considerable interobserver variation.

Symptoms and signs are useful in alerting the clinician to the possibility of heart failure. The diagnosis, however, must be supported by further tests [72] (Table 5.12). These should be geared towards assessing cardiac function and

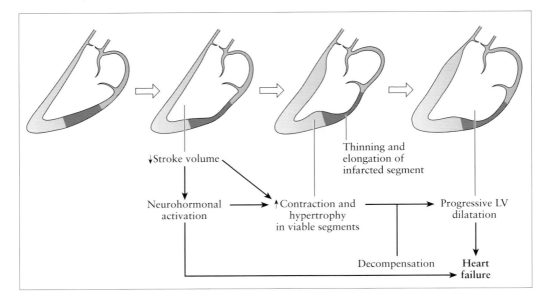

Figure 5.5 Pathophysiology of left ventricular (LV) dysfunction following myocardial infarction. Following a myocardial infarction, the infarcted segment loses tensile strength and becomes increasingly incapable of withstanding the ventricular systolic load imposed by hypertension. The infarcted segment thins and elongates, and may become aneurysmal or even rupture. More frequently, a non-distensible fibrous scar forms. Immediate reductions in stroke volume cause neurohormonal activation, such as sympatho-adrenal activation, which increases heart rate and the force of ventricular contraction in viable segments. Reduced systolic contraction leads to incomplete ventricular emptying and thus, elevations in LV end-diastolic pressure, which causes increased diastolic wall stress. As well as causing distortion and distension of the previously infarcted segment, increased LV wall stress also causes compensatory hypertrophy of viable myocardium. The combined effect of these processes is to 'remodel' the LV. Although LV remodelling could be regarded as compensatory, it becomes uncompensated in ≈ 40% of patients. The result is a persistent increase in LV wall stress, neurohormonal activation, progressive reductions in stroke volume and the clinical features of heart failure.

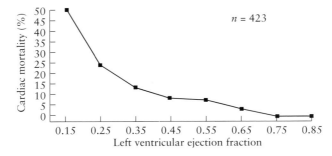

Figure 5.6 The relationship between left ventricular ejection fraction and 1-year cardiac mortality after myocardial infarction. Reproduced from [69] with permission of WB Saunders Co. Ltd, London, UK.

Table 5.11 Characteristics of hypertensive patients with heart failure.

	Men	Women
Age	73 ± 9	78 ± 9
Blood pressure (mmHg)		
systolic	149 ± 21	150 ± 22
diastolic	81 ± 13	77 ± 12
Previous history of*:		
Myocardial infarction (%)	52	34
Angina (%)†	48	56
Diabetes mellitus (%)	24	28
ECG — Left ventricular hypertrophy (%)	21	23
Valvular heart disease (%)	24	33

Analysis of 165 men and 192 women. The diagnosis of heart failure was made on the basis of clinical criteria. The diagnosis of diabetes was defined on the basis of a fasting blood glucose of > 7.77 mmol l^{-1} (140 mg dl^{-1}), two random non-fasting levels > 11.1 mmol l^{-1} (200 mg dl^{-1}) or the use of insulin or oral hypoglycaemics. Results presented as mean SD or in the case of*, in %.
†With or without a previous myocardial infarction.
Adapted from [69].

Table 5.12 Investigations for patients with heart failure.

Routine investigations
FBC
U+Es, creatinine, glucose, calcium and albumin
TSH in patients with AF or unexplained heart failure
Urinalysis for micro- and macroalbuminuria
Chest X-ray
ECG
Transthoracic echocardiogram

Targeted investigations
Radionuclide ventriculography to assess left ventricular function
Non-invasive stress testing to detect ischaemia:
    In patients without angina but with a high probability of CHD who would be candidates for revascularization
    To assess myocardial viability or coronary arteriography in patients with a previous infarction but with no angina who would be candidates for revascularization
Coronary arteriography in patients with angina or large areas of ischaemic or hibernating myocardium; also in patients at risk for coronary artery disease who are to undergo surgical correction of non-coronary cardiac lesions.
Ambulatory blood pressure monitoring in patients with heart failure who have borderline elevations in blood pressure

TSH, thyroid stimulating hormone; AF, atrial fibrillation.

at excluding other conditions which masquerade as or exacerbate heart failure (Table 5.13) [72]. Once the diagnosis has been established, the New York Heart Association (NYHA) classification (Table 5.14) is useful in grading the severity of heart failure and the response to treatment.

Table 5.13 Conditions which masquerade as or exacerbate heart failure.

Lung disease
Anaemia
Renal or hepatic disease
Reversible myocardial ischaemia

Table 5.14 The New York Heart Association (NYHA) classification of heart failure.

Class I*	No limitation: ordinary physical exercise does not cause undue fatigue, dyspnoea or palpitations
Class II	Slight limitation of physical activity: comfortable at rest but ordinary activity results in fatigue, palpitations, dyspnoea or angina
Class III	Marked limitation of physical activity: comfortable at rest but less than ordinary physical activity results in symptoms
Class IV	Unable to carry out any physical activity without discomfort: symptoms of heart failure are present even at rest with increased discomfort with any physical activity

*Patients in Class I would have to have objective evidence of cardiac dysfunction, a history of heart failure symptoms or a history of treatment for heart failure.

Special investigations

Cardiac dysfunction has been classically equated with impaired ventricular contraction, i.e. systolic dysfunction. It is well recognized, however, that up to 40% of patients with symptoms of heart failure have normal systolic function [73]. Disorders of ventricular relaxation, i.e. diastolic dysfunction, can occur before the development of overt cardiac failure, in patients with normal systolic function and in those without LVH. The occurrence of diastolic dysfunction before systolic dysfunction is a characteristic early feature of hypertensive heart failure.

Echocardiography. This is dealt with on p. 32.

Exercise testing. A normal treadmill exercise test in a patient not receiving heart failure treatment excludes the diagnosis. In patients with established heart failure, exercise testing may add to the assessment of severity and to monitoring progress and response to treatment. Cardiopulmonary assessment, comprising measurement of oxygen consumption and carbon dioxide production during exercise, may be useful in the diagnosis of heart failure.

Other tests. Nuclear angiography provides a measure of global left and right ventricular systolic function, but does not evaluate valve function, regional wall motion abnormalities or ventricular hypertrophy. It should, therefore, be reserved for patients in whom echocardiography is not possible.

Treatment

Numerous studies have shown that antihypertensive treatment prevents the development of heart failure [74–76] and that treatment of cardiac failure *per se* improves survival [73,77–79]. The pharmacological treatment of heart failure and left ventricular dysfunction is outlined in Table 5.15 and Fig. 5.7.

ACE inhibitors. Although no studies have specifically assessed the impact on mortality of ACE inhibitors in patients with hypertensive heart failure, their effectiveness in reducing mortality, delaying progression of ventricular dilatation and left ventricular dysfunction following MI is undoubted. Importantly, the benefits in terms of lives saved are superior to other medical treatments (Table 5.16). The benefits are not only seen in patients who have shown signs of heart failure, but also in those with asymptomatic left ventricular dysfunction. In the light of these findings, ACE inhibitors should be considered in all hypertensive patients who have had signs of heart failure or left ventricular systolic dysfunction (ejection fraction of < 0.40 on echocardiography, radionuclide scans or LV angiography), regardless of whether or not they have had an MI. The apparent reluctance [80–82] to prescribe these cost-effective [82] agents in patients with heart failure is unjustified, even in the light of perceived problems with first-dose and postural hypotension and renal function. In the light of the relative costs of ACE inhibitor treatment for heart failure (Table 5.17), a public health system can ill-afford *not* to prescribe them for this purpose.

Table 5.15 Recommended pharmacological therapy for patients with chronic heart failure.

- ACE inhibitors *indefinitely* at optimum doses for all patients with:
  Symptomatic heart failure
  Objective signs of heart failure at any time
  Asymptomatic left ventricular dysfunction (ejection fraction < 0.40)
- Loop diuretics (frusemide, bumetanide) for patients with fluid overload*
- Hydralazine and nitrates in patients who are intolerant of ACE inhibitors
- Digoxin for patients with:
  AF and rapid ventricular rates
  Heart failure not responding to ACE inhibitors and diuretics†
- β-blockers under specialist supervision
- Anticoagulation in patients with:
  AF, or
  Previous systemic or pulmonary embolism
- Specific lipid-lowering therapy with statins in patients with CHD

Calcium channel blockers, with the possible exception of amlodipine, are not recommended in systolic heart failure. Low dose dobutamine or milrinone infusion has been used with some success in selected patients with refractory heart failure, but these agents shorten survival.
*Therapy with loop diuretics should be used in conjunction with ACE inhibitors and will need to be maintained even when the patient is free of oedema. This will require dose titration.
†Digoxin may be beneficial in heart failure from systolic dysfunction, but it probably does not improve survival.

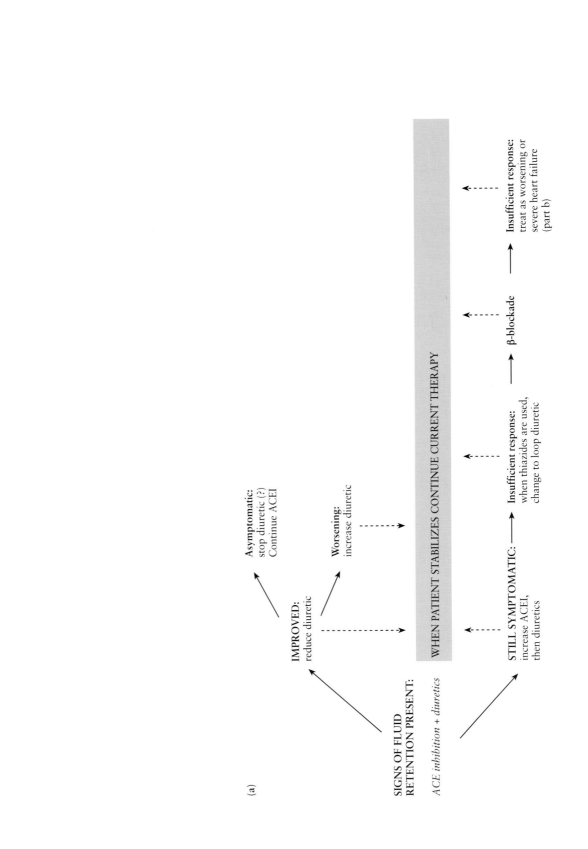

(a)

SIGNS OF FLUID
RETENTION PRESENT:

ACE inhibition + diuretics

IMPROVED:
reduce diuretic

Asymptomatic:
stop diuretic (?)
Continue ACEI

Worsening:
increase diuretic

STILL SYMPTOMATIC:
increase ACEI,
then diuretics

Insufficient response:
when thiazides are used,
change to loop diuretic

β-blockade

Insufficient response:
treat as worsening or
severe heart failure
(part b)

WHEN PATIENT STABILIZES CONTINUE CURRENT THERAPY

(b)

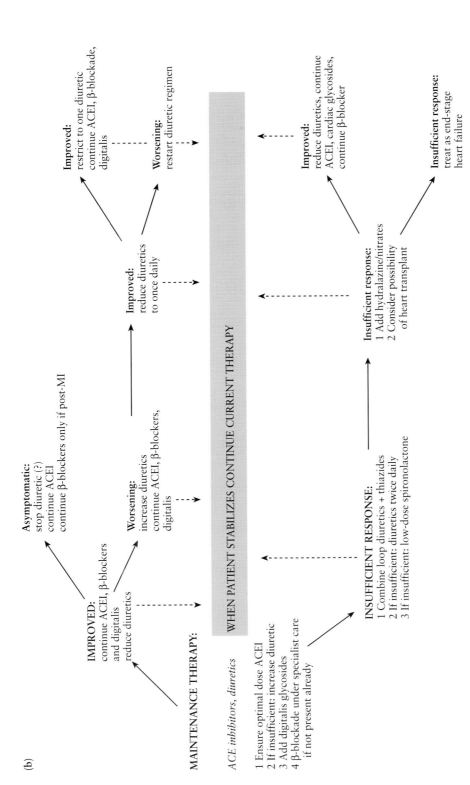

Asymptomatic:
stop diuretic (?)
continue ACEI
continue β-blockers only if post-MI

Worsening:
restart diuretic regimen

Improved:
restrict to one diuretic
continue ACEI, β-blockade,
digitalis

IMPROVED:
continue ACEI, β-blockers
and digitalis
reduce diuretics

Worsening:
increase diuretics
continue ACEI, β-blockers,
digitalis

Improved:
reduce diuretics
to once daily

Improved:
reduce diuretics, continue
ACEI, cardiac glycosides,
continue β-blocker

MAINTENANCE THERAPY:

WHEN PATIENT STABILIZES CONTINUE CURRENT THERAPY

ACE inhibitors, diuretics

1 Ensure optimal dose ACEI
2 If insufficient: increase diuretic
3 Add digitalis glycosides
4 β-blockade under specialist care
   if not present already

INSUFFICIENT RESPONSE:
1 Combine loop diuretics + thiazides
2 If insufficient: diuretics twice daily
3 If insufficient: low-dose spironolactone

Insufficient response:
1 Add hydralazine/nitrates
2 Consider possibility
   of heart transplant

Insufficient response:
treat as end-stage
heart failure

Figure 5.7 Steps in the management of heart failure. Reproduced from [72] with permission of WB Saunders Co. Ltd, London, UK.

Table 5.16 Comparative benefits of ACE inhibitors in heart failure.

Treatment	Events prevented per 1000 patient-years of treatment
ACEI for severe heart failure	160 deaths
ACEI for mild/moderate heart failure	16 deaths, 3 MIs — unstable angina, 116 hospitalizations
ACEI after MI (low LVEF, as in SAVE study)	12 deaths, 9 MIs, 16 heart failure, 10 revascularizations
Diuretic/β-blocker for mild hypertension	1–2 strokes
Aspirin after MI	16 deaths / MIs / strokes
Oral β-blockers after MI	13 deaths, 5 MIs
Statins after MI or angina	6 deaths, 12 MIs, 4 heart failure, 11 revascularizations

ACEI, ACE inhibitor; MI, myocardial infarction; LVEF, left ventricular ejection fraction.
Adapted from [83].

Table 5.17 Cost of various medical treatments*.

Treatment	Cost (£)†
ACE inhibitor for mild-to-moderate CHF‡	502
Pacemaker implant	1100
Valve replacement for aortic stenosis	1140
Hip replacement	1180
CABG (left main stem stenosis+severe angina)	2090
Kidney transplant	4710
Breast cancer screening	5780
Heart transplant	7840
CABG (single vessel disease+moderate angina)	18 830
Hospital haemodyalisis	21 970

*For the year 1990.
†Cost per quality adjusted life for various medical treatments.
‡Treatment initiated in 40% one-day inpatients and 60% in general practice (i.e. in the community).
CABG, coronary artery bypass grafting.
Reproduced from [84] with permission of Adis International Ltd, Auckland, New Zealand.

Doses. The possibility of first-dose hypotension needs to be addressed (p. 186). To achieve the maximum benefit, ACE inhibitors should be titrated to optimum doses (Table 5.18). After MI, ACE inhibitors should be commenced once the patient is stable post-thrombolysis and the target should be to reach the optimum dose within 7 days. Care should be taken to avoid hypotension and that the plasma creatinine does not rise by > 20 μmol l^{-1}.

Other agents. β-blocker therapy in heart failure appears promising, both in terms of symptom control and in reduction of mortality [85–87]. Carvedilol [88] and bisoprolol are notable in this respect. In the ELITE study of patients with heart failure aged > 65 years, treatment with the angiotensin receptor

Table 5.18 Target doses for treatment of heart failure with ACE inhibitors.

Drug	Target dose	Study
Captopril	50 mg b.d./t.d.s.	ISIS-4, SAVE
Ramipril	5 mg b.d.	AIRE
Enalapril	10–20 mg b.d.	VHeFT II, CONSENSUS
Trandolapril	4 mg o.d.	TRACE
Zofenopril	30 mg b.d.	SMILE
Lisinopril	10 mg o.d.	GISSI-3

antagonist losartan was associated with an unexpectedly lower mortality than that found with captopril [89]. This should be taken into account in patients with heart failure who develop a cough with ACE inhibitors.

VALVULAR DISEASE: AORTIC STENOSIS AND REGURGITATION

Systemic hypertension not only affects the myocardium and the coronary vasculature but also the heart valves (Fig. 5.8), particularly in patients with pre-existing valvular heart disease, such as aortic stenosis, aortic regurgitation and mitral regurgitation. In these patients, early detection of hypertension and its adequate control is paramount.

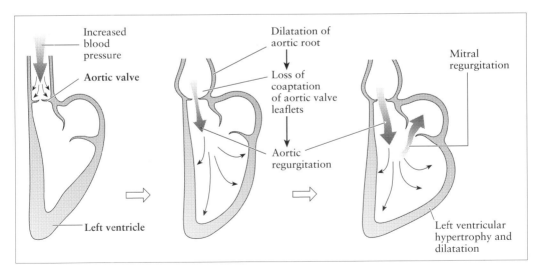

Figure 5.8 Pathophysiology of aortic valve disease in hypertension. Systemic hypertension leads to dilatation of the aortic root and disruption of the three-dimensional arrangement of the aortic valve within the aortic root. Loss of coaption and distortion of valve leaflets lead to regurgitation of some of the ejected volume back into the left ventricle (LV), thus increasing end-diastolic pressure, which contributes to left ventricular hypertrophy and dilatation. As the ventricle dilates, the three-dimensional arrangement of the mitral valve apparatus is disrupted, leading to mitral regurgitation.

Diagnosis

The detection of aortic stenosis in hypertensive patients is important because vasodilators, especially ACE inhibitors, can precipitate acute renal failure. This is related to reduced renal perfusion caused by the combination of increased peripheral vasodilatation and a critical obstruction to left ventricular outflow.

Aortic stenosis and regurgitation should be considered in patients with reduced exercise tolerance or dyspnoea at rest. The volume and character of the radial pulse and auscultatory findings may support the diagnosis. Aortic stenosis should also be suspected in patients whose plasma creatinine rises by > 20 µmol l⁻¹ whilst on treatment with vasodilators, especially ACE inhibitors. It should be noted, however, that renal artery stenosis is more often the culprit of ACE-induced elevations in plasma creatinine levels.

Treatment. The treatment of critical aortic stenosis and aortic regurgitation is aortic valve replacement. In both aortic stenosis and aortic regurgitation, systolic blood pressures should be kept < 140 mmHg.

1 *Aortic stenosis*: β-blockers, by increasing diastolic filling time and improving the function of a stiff, hypertrophied ventricle, may be advantageous. ACE inhibitors should be avoided in patients with significant aortic stenosis (when the peak transaortic gradient > 40 mmHg), because of the danger of precipitating profound hypotension, renal failure and myocardial ischaemia, especially if there is co-existing CHD. If ACE inhibitors are considered paramount, a cardiology opinion should be sought.

2 *Aortic regurgitation*: Because of their capacity to retard the progression and delay the need for surgical intervention [90], ACE inhibitors are considered as first choice. Similar effects occur with dihydropyridine calcium antagonists [91] and with hydralazine [92]. β-Blockers should be used with caution in severe aortic regurgitation with attending left ventricular failure.

CARDIAC ARRHYTHMIAS

Cardiac arrhythmias in hypertensive patients are related to the hypertensive process, to associated CHD and to the neurohormonal disturbances that are commonly associated with these conditions, notably sympathetic nervous system activation. Myocardial fibrosis, resulting from LVH and/or CHD (either macro- or microvascular), facilitates re-entrant arrhythmias and reduces the threshold for ventricular fibrillation.

Sustained ventricular arrhythmias

These are probably the commonest cause of sudden death in hypertensive patients. The risk of sudden death in hypertensive patients increases in proportion to blood pressure levels [93] and to the presence of ventricular

ectopy, LVH and left ventricular dysfunction. Patients with sustained ventricular arrhythmias should be referred to the cardiologist.

Ventricular ectopy

As discussed above, attempts at suppressing ventricular ectopy in survivors
of MI have either been shown to increase mortality or to be ineffective.
β-Blockers are the only anti-arrhythmic drugs that have so far been shown to
improve prognosis in post-MI patients. Amiodarone should be considered in
patients with impaired LV function and multifocal ventricular ectopy. Such
cases should be referred to a cardiologist.

Atrial fibrillation (AF)

AF occurs commonly in hypertensive patients, and contributes to considerable morbidity and mortality. Up to 15% of strokes are preceded by AF [94].
It is more frequent in the elderly and in patients with structural heart disease.
At the outset, patients may experience palpitations and, less commonly,
fatigue, dyspnoea and dizziness, but usually patients are asymptomatic. The
ECG is characteristic (Fig. 5.9). Detailed management recommendations are
available [95,96].

The three aspects to the management of patients with AF, with or without
hypertension, are as follows:

Restoration and maintenance of sinus rhythm. Cardioversion should be considered if there is a reasonable chance that the patient will remain in sinus
rhythm long term. The probability of remaining in sinus rhythm diminishes if
AF has persisted for more than 12 months, if the atria are dilated (left atrial
dimension on echocardiography of > 4 cm) or if there are other promoting
factors, such as mitral valve disease. Direct current (DC) cardioversion
should be considered in patients who are haemodynamically compromised
or alternatively, as an elective procedure. Pharmacological cardioversion and
maintenance of sinus rhythm with procainamide, amiodarone, quinidine,
disopyramide, sotalol and propafenone may also be considered. Intravenous digoxin does not increase the rate of conversion to sinus rhythm
[97,98].

Control of ventricular rate. Uncontrolled ventricular rates may lead to
symptoms and to tachycardia-induced cardiomyopathy. For long-term
control, β-blockers are the drugs of choice, because they are effective at
controlling both blood pressure and the ventricular response. Digoxin is
less effective, but should be considered as first choice in patients with left
ventricular dysfunction. Combinations of digoxin, β-blockers and either
verapamil or diltiazem may be needed for effective control of the ventricular
response.

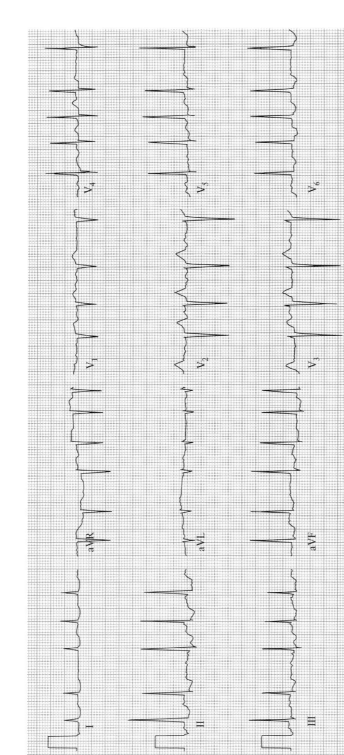

Figure 5.9 ECG of a patient with atrial fibrillation. Note the unco-ordinated atrial rate, characterized by the absence of P waves and an irregular baseline. The ventricular rate is characteristically irregular and unless there is co-existent ventricular disease, the QRS complex is unaffected. It is important not to overlook abnormalities of the QRS complex, as these may indicate underlying coronary heart disease or left ventricular hypertrophy. In this case, there is ST-segment depression in most leads, suggesting myocardial ischaemia.

Table 5.19 Indications for anticoagulation in chronic atrial fibrillation*.

Clinical indications
Age (alone) > 65 years [109]
Previous stroke, TIA or peripheral embolic event†
Hypertension [109]
Diabetes [109]
Dilated cardiomyopathy

Echocardiographic indications
Mitral stenosis
Left atrial dilatation > 40 mm [110,111]
Impaired left ventricular function‡ [110–114]
Mitral annular calcification [115]
'Unstable' intraventricular thrombus§
Patent foramen ovale [116,117]
Atrial septal aneurysm [118]

---

*In our view, all patients < 65 years with chronic atrial fibrillation who, in addition, have at least one of the above risk factors should receive anticoagulation, unless contra-indicated.
†Includes a renal embolic event.
‡Currently debated.
§Non-organized intraventricular thrombus which is seen to protrude into the ventricular cavity on echocardiography.

Prevention of thrombo-embolism. Patients with AF are at an increased risk of cerebral and systemic embolization [99–106]. At autopsy, 30–40% and up to 70% of patients who have had AF have peripheral and cerebral emboli, respectively.

There is now overwhelming evidence indicating that long-term anti-coagulant treatment prevents cerebrovascular disease in patients with AF. Warfarin treatment, maintaining international normalized ratio (INR) between 1.8 and 4.2, has been shown to reduce the risk of thrombo-embolic stroke associated with AF by almost 70%, with low-dose anticoagulation conferring much less benefit. One should be aware of high discontinuation rates [100] and higher risk of haemorrhage in patients > 75 years, in whom INR levels should be monitored very closely. Unless contra-indicated, warfarin (to maintain a target INR of 3.0) should always be considered mandatory in patients with AF who have had a stroke, a transient ischaemic attack or peripheral embolism. Adequate blood pressure control must be achieved before committing hypertensive patients to anticoagulant therapy. Indications for warfarin treatment in patients with chronic AF are shown in Table 5.19. The currently recommended targets for INR in anticoagulant therapy are shown in Table 5.20.

Note: Aspirin appears to prevent non-cardioembolic stroke, but does not prevent cardioembolic strokes [107,108]. It should therefore be reserved for patients with contra-indications to warfarin and for young subjects without additional risk factors for cardioembolic stroke. Dipyridamole has not been evaluated in patients with AF.

Table 5.20 Recommended international normalized ratio (INR) during treatment with warfarin, according to condition predisposing to embolism.

Condition	Recommended range of INR*
Atrial fibrillation	
> 75 years	2.0–2.5†
Non-rheumatic AF	2.0–3.0
+ Previous stroke or TIA	2.0–3.9
+ Mechanical valve prosthesis	3.0–4.5

*The aim of treatment should be to keep the INR from falling below or rising above the indicated limits. INR levels below 2.0 are associated with much higher levels of stroke and therefore, 'low-dose' regimens are no longer recommended [119, 120].
†A lower target because of the increased risk of haemorrhage in this age group.

References

1   Kannel WB, Stokes J. Hypertension as a cardiovascular risk factor. In: Birkenhager W, Reid J, eds. *Handbook of Hypertension*, Vol. 6. Amsterdam: Elsevier, 1985: 15–34.

2   Kannel WB, Belanger AJ. Epidemiology of heart failure. *Am Heart J* 1991; 121: 951–957.

3   Neaton JD, Wentworth D. Serum cholesterol, blood pressure, cigarette smoking, and death from coronary artery disease: overall findings and differences by age for 316 099 white men: Multiple Risk Factor Intervention Trial (MRFIT). *Arch Intern Med* 1992; 152: 56–64.

4   The Coronary Drug Project Research Group. Blood pressure in survivors of myocardial infarction. *J Am Coll Cardiol* 1984; 4: 1134.

5   DeBusk RF, Kraemer HC, Nash E. Stepwise risk stratification soon after myocardial infarction. *Am J Cardiol* 1983; 52: 1161.

6   Merrilees MA, Scott PJ, Norris RM. Prognosis after myocardial infarction: results of 15 year follow-up. *BMJ* 1984; 288: 356.

7   Maisel AS, Gilpin E, Holt B *et al.* Survival after hospital discharge in matched populations with inferior and anterior myocardial infarction. *J Am Coll Cardiol* 1985; 6: 631.

8   Luscher TF. The endothelium in hypertension: bystander, target or mediator? *J Hum Hypertens* 1994; 12 (Suppl.): S105–106.

9   Bean WB. Masquerade of myocardial infarction. *Lancet* 1977; 1: 1044.

10 Shaper AG, Cook DG, Walker J, Mcfarlane PW. Prevalence of ischaemic heart disease in middle aged British men. *Br Heart J* 1984; 51: 595–605.

11 Margolis JR, Kannel WB, Feinlieb M *et al.* Clinical features of unrecognized myocardial infarction: Silent and symptomatic. Eighteen year follow up. The Framingham Study. *Am J Cardiol* 1973; 32: 1.

12 Daly LE, Lonergan M, Graham I. Predicting operative mortality after coronary artery bypass surgery in males. *Quart J Med* 1993; 68: 771–778.

13 Vogt M, Motz W, Schwartzkopff B, Strauer BE. Coronary microangiopathy and cardiac hypertrophy. *Eur Heart J* 1990; 1 (Suppl. B): 133–138.

14 Houghton JL, Frank MJ, Carr AA, von Dohlen TW, Prisant LM. Relations among impaired coronary flow reserve, left ventricular hypertrophy and thallium perfusion defects in hypertensive patients without obstructive coronary artery disease. *J Am Coll Cardiol* 1990; 15: 43–51.

15 Weissler AM. Exercise testing. *Circulation* 1977; 56: 699.

16 Weiner DA, Ryan TJ, McCabe CH *et al.* Exercise stress testing. Correlations among history of angina, ST-segment response and prevalence of coronary-artery disease in the coronary artery surgery study (CASS). *N Engl J Med* 1979; 301: 203–205.

17 Diamond GA, Forrester JS. Analysis of probability as an aid in the clinical diagnosis of coronary artery disease. *N Engl J Med* 1979; 300: 1350–1358.

18 North of England Stable Angina Guideline Development Group. North of England evidence based guidelines development project: summary, Version of evidence based guideline for the primary care management of stable angina. *BMJ* 1996; 312: 827–832.

19 Beevers DG, Johnston JH, Larkin H, Davies P. Clinical evidence that β-adrenoceptor blockers prevent more cardiovascular complications than other anti-hypertensive drugs. *Drugs* 1983; 25 (Suppl.): 326–330.

20 Nidorf SM, Thompson PL, Jamrozik KD, Hobbs MST. Reduced risk of death at 28 days in patients taking β-blocker before admission to hospital with myocardial infarction. *BMJ* 1990; 300: 71–74.

21 Psaty BM, Koepsell TD, Wagner EH, LoGerfo JP, Inui TS. The relative risk of incident coronary heart disease associated with recently stopping the use of β-blockers. *JAMA* 1990; 263: 1653–1657.

22 Meluzin J, Zeman K, Steka P, Simek P. Effects of nifedipine and diltiazem on myocardial ischemia in patients with severe stable angina pectoris treated with nitrates and β-blockers. *J Cardiovasc Pharmacol* 1992; 20: 864–869.

23 Woodmansey PA, Stewart G, Morice AH, Channer KS. Amlodipine in patients with angina uncontrolled by atenolol. A double blind placebo controlled cross over trial. *Eur J Clin Pharmacol* 1993; 45: 107–111.

24 Fox KM, Muchany D, Findlay I, Ford I, Dargie HJ. Group on behalf of the TIBET Study. The Total Ischaemic Burden European Trial (TIBET). Effects of atenolol, nifedipine SR and their combination on the exercise test and the total ischaemic burden in 608 patients with stable angina. *Eur Heart J* 1996; 17: 96–103.

25 McMurray J. Reductions in mortality post-myocardial infarction: recent clinical trial data. *Br J Cardiol* 1995; 2 (Suppl. 2): S15–S17.

26 ISIS-2 (Second International Study of Infarct Survival) Collaborative Group. Randomized trial of intravenous streptokinase, oral aspirin, both or neither among 17 187 cases of suspected acute myocardial infarction: ISIS-2. *Lancet* 1988; 2: 349–360.

27 Juul-Moller S, Edvardsson N, Jahnmatz B *et al.* Double-blind trial of aspirin in primary prevention of myocardial infarction in patients with stable chronic angina pectoris. *Lancet* 1992; 340: 1421–1425.

28 Lewis HD, Davis JW, Archibald DG *et al.* Protective effects of aspirin against acute myocardial infarction and death in men with unstable angina: results of a Veterans Administration cooperative study. *N Engl J Med* 1983; 309: 396–403.

29 Wallentin LC. Aspirin (75 mg/day) after an episode of unstable coronary artery disease: long-term effects on the risk for myocardial infarction, occurrence of severe angina and the need for revascularization. *J Am Coll Cardiol* 1991; 18: 1587–1593.

30 The Salt Collaborative Group. Swedish aspirin low-dose trial (SALT) of 75 mg aspirin as secondary prophylaxis after cerebrovascular ischemic events. *Lancet* 1991; 338: 1345–1349.

31 The Dutch TIA Trial Study Group. A comparison of two doses of aspirin (30 mg vs 283 mg a day) in patients after a transient ischemic attack or minor ischemic stroke. *N Engl J Med* 1991; 325: 1261–1266.

32   Nyman I, Larsson H, Wallentin L. Prevention of serious cardiac events by low-dose aspirin in patients with silent myocardial ischemia. *Lancet* 1992; 340: 497–501.

33   Antiplatelet Trialists' Collaboration. Collaborative overview of randomized trials of anti-platelet therapy. I. Prevention of death, myocardial infarction and stroke by prolonged anti-platelet therapy in various categories of patients. *BMJ* 1994; 308: 81–106.

34   Antiplatelet Trialists' Collaboration. Secondary prevention of vascular disease by prolonged anti-platelet treatment. *BMJ* 1988; 296: 320–331.

35   Antiplatelet Trialists' Collaboration. Collaborative overview of randomized trials of antiplatelet therapy. II. Maintenance of vascular graft or arterial patency by antiplatelet therapy. *BMJ* 1994; 308: 159–168.

36   Antiplatelet Trialists' Collaboration. Collaborative overview of randomized trials of antiplatelet therapy. III. Reduction in venous thrombosis and pulmonary embolism by antiplatelet prophylaxis among surgical and medical patients. *BMJ* 1994; 308: 235–246.

37   Frishman WH, Furberg DC, Friedewald WT. β-adrenergic blockade for survivors of acute myocardial infarction. *N Engl J Med* 1984; 310: 830–836.

38   Yusuf S, Wittes J, Friedman L. Overview of results of randomized clinical trials in heart disease: treatment following myocardial infarction. *JAMA* 1988; 260: 2088–2093.

39   Norwegian Multicentre Study Group. Timolol-induced reduction in mortality and reinfarction in patients surviving acute myocardial infarction. *N Engl J Med* 1981; 304: 801–807.

40   β-Blocker Heart Attack Trial Research Group. A randomized trial of propanolol in patients with acute myocardial infarction. I. Mortality results. *JAMA* 1982; 247: 1707–1714.

41   MIAMI Trial Research Group. Metoprolol in acute myocardial infarction (MIAMI). A randomized placebo-controlled international trial. *Eur Heart J* 1985; 6: 199–226.

42   ISIS-I (First International Study of Infarct Survival) Collaborative Group. Randomized trial of intravenous atenolol among 16 027 cases of suspected acute myocardial infarction. ISIS-I. *Lancet* 1986; ii: 57–66.

43   Roberts R, Rogers WJ, Mueller HS *et al.* Immediate versus deferred β-blockade following thrombolytic therapy in patients with acute myocardial infarction: results of the Thrombolysis In Acute Myocardial Infarction (TIMI) ii-B subgroup analysis. *Circulation* 1991; 83: 422–437.

44   Psaty BM, Heckbert SR, Koepsell TD *et al.* The risk of myocardial infarction associated with antihypertensive agents. *JAMA* 1995; 274: 620–625.

45   American College of Cardiology. American Heart Association. Guidelines for the management of patients with acute myocardial infarction: a report of the ACC/AHA Task Force on Practice Guidelines (Committee on Management of Acute Myocardial Infarction). *J Am Coll Cardiol* 1996; 28: 1328–1419.

46   Scandinavian Simvastatin Survival Study Group. Randomized trial of cholesterol lowering in 4444 patients with coronary heart disease: the Scandinavian Simvastatin Survival Study (4S). *Lancet* 1994; 344: 1383–1389.

47   Sacks FM, Pfeffer MA, Moye LA *et al.* The effect of pravastatin on coronary events after myocardial infarction in patients with average cholesterol levels. *N Engl J Med* 1996; 335: 1001–1009.

48   The Long Term Intervention with Pravastatin in Ischemic Disease (LIPID) Study Group. Prevention of cardiovascular events and death with pravastatin in patients

with coronary heart disease and a broad range of initial cholesterol levels. *New Engl J Med* 1999; 339: 1349–1357.

49 Byington RP, Jukema JW, Salonen JT *et al.* Reduction in cardiovascular events during pravastatin therapy: pooled analysis of clinical events of the pravastatin atherosclerosis intervention program. *Circulation* 1995; 92: 2419–2425.

50 Casale PN, Devereux RB, Milner M *et al.* Value of echocardiographic measurement of left ventricular mass in predicting cardiovascular morbid events in hypertensive men. *Ann Intern Med* 1986; 105: 173–178.

51 Levy D, Garrison RJ, Savage DD *et al.* Prognostic implications of echocardiographically determined left ventricular mass in the Framingham Heart Study. *N Engl J Med* 1990; 322: 1561–1566.

52 Koren MJ, Devereux RB, Casale PN *et al.* Relation of left ventricular mass and geometry to morbidity and mortality in uncomplicated essential hypertension. *Ann Intern Med* 1991; 114: 345–352.

53 Kannel WB, Levy D, Cupples LA. Left ventricular hypertrophy and risk of cardiac failure: insights from the Framingham Study. *J Cardiovasc Pharmacol* 1987; 10 (Suppl. 6): S135–S140.

54 Kannel WB. Prevalence and natural history of electrocardiographic left ventricular hypertrophy. *Am J Med* 1983; 75: 4–11.

55 Bolognese L, Dellavesa P, Rossi L *et al.* Prognostic value of left ventricular mass in uncomplicated acute myocardial infarction and one-vessel coronary artery disease. *Am J Cardiol* 1994; 73: 1–5.

56 Boden WE, Kleiger RE, Schechtman KB *et al.* Clinical significance and prognostic importance of left ventricular hypertrophy in non-Q-wave acute myocardial infarction. *Am J Cardiol* 1988; 62: 1000–1004.

57 Liao Y, Cooper RS, McGee DL *et al.* The relative effects of left ventricular hypertrophy, coronary artery disease, and ventricular dysfunction on survival among black adults. *JAMA* 1995; 273: 1592–1597.

58 Cosin Aguilar J, Hernandiz Martinez A, Andres Conejos F. Mechanisms of ventricular arrhythmias in the presence of pathological hypertrophy. *Eur Heart J* 1993; 14 (Suppl. J): 65–70.

59 Schmieder RE, Martus P, Klingbeil A. Reversal of left ventricular hypertrophy in essential hypertension — a metaanalysis of randomized double-blind studies. *JAMA* 1996; 275: 1507–1513.

60 Dahlöf P, Pennert K, Hansson L. Reversal of left ventricular hypertrophy in hypertensive patients: a metaanalysis of 109 treatment studies. *Am J Hypertens* 1992; 5: 95–110.

61 Liebson PR. Clinical studies of drug reversal of hypertensive left ventricular hypertrophy. *Am J Hypertens* 1990; 3: 512–517.

62 Muiesan ML, Salvetti M, Rizzoni D *et al.* Association of change in left-ventricular mass with prognosis during long-term antihypertensive treatment. *J Hypertens* 1995; 13: 1091–1095.

63 Linzbach AJ. Heart failure from the point of view of quantitative anatomy. *Am J Cardiol* 1960; 5: 370–382.

64 Agabiti-Rosei E, Ambrosini E, Dal Palù C *et al.* on behalf of the RACE Study Group. ACE inhibitor ramipril is more effective than β-blocker atenolol in reducing left ventricular mass in hypertension. Results of the RACE (Ramipril Cardioprotective Evaluation) study. *J Hypertens* 1995; 13: 1325–1335.

65 Kannel WB, Castelli WP, McNamara PM, McKee PA, Feinlieb M. Role of blood pressure in the development of congestive heart failure: the Framingham Study. *N Engl J Med* 1972; 287: 781–787.

66   Eriksson H, Svardsudd K, Larsson B *et al.* Risk factors for heart failure in the general population: the study of men born in 1913. *Eur Heart J* 1989; 10: 647–677.

67   Kannel WB, Ho K, Thom T. Changing epidemiologic features of cardiac failure. *Br Heart J* 1994; 72 (Suppl.): 3–9.

68   Gadsboll N, Hoilund-Carlsen PF, Madsen EB *et al.* Right and left ventricular ejection fractions: relation to one-year prognosis in acute myocardial infarction. *Eur Heart J* 1987; 8: 1201–1209.

69   Levy E, Larson MG, Ramachandran SV, Kannel WB, Ho KKL. The progression from hypertension to congestive heart failure. *JAMA* 1996; 275: 1557–1562.

70   Butman SM, Ewy GA, Standen JR, Kern KB, Hahn E. Bedside cardiovascular examination in patients with severe chronic heart failure. *J Am Coll Cardiol* 1993; 22: 968–974.

71   Stevenson LW, Perloff JK. The limited reliability of physical signs for estimating hemodynamics in chronic heart failure. *JAMA* 1989; 261: 884–888.

72   The Task Force on Heart Failure of the European Society of Cardiology. Guidelines for the diagnosis of heart failure. *Eur Heart J* 1995; 16: 741–751.

73   The SOLVD Investigators. Effect of enalapril on mortality and development of heart failure in asymptomatic patients with reduced left ventricular ejection fraction. *N Engl J Med* 1992; 327: 685–691.

74   Veterans Administration Cooperative Study Group on Antihypertensive Agents. Effects of treatment on morbidity in hypertension: results in patients with diastolic blood pressures averaging 115 through 129 mmHg. *JAMA* 1967; 202: 1028–1034.

75   Veterans Administration Cooperative Study Group on Antihypertensive Agents. Effects of treatment on morbidity in hypertension, II. results in patients with diastolic blood pressures averaging 90 through 114 mmHg. *JAMA* 1970; 213: 1143–1151.

76   SHEP Cooperative Research Group. Prevention of stroke by antihypertensive drug treatment in older persons with isolated systolic hypertension: final results of the Systolic Hypertension in the Elderly Program (SHEP). *JAMA* 1991; 265: 3255–3264.

77   Pfeffer MA, Braunwald E, Moye LA *et al.* Effect of captopril on mortality and morbidity in patients with left ventricular dysfunction after myocardial infarction: results of the Survival and Ventricular enlargement Trial. *N Engl J Med* 1992; 327: 669–677.

78   Acute Infarction Ramipril Efficacy (AIRE) Investigators. Effects of ramipril on mortality and morbidity of survivors of acute myocardial infarction with clinical evidence of heart failure. *Lancet* 1993; 324: 821–828.

79   Kober L, Torp-Pederson C, Carlsen JE *et al.* A clinical trial of the angiotensin-converting enzyme inhibitor tandolapril in patients with left ventricular dysfunction after myocardial infarction. *N Engl J Med* 1995; 333: 1670–1676.

80   Hart W, Rhodes G, McMurray J. The cost-effectiveness of enalapril in the treatment of chronic heart failure. *Br J Med Economics* 1993; 6: 91–98.

81   Mair FS, Crowley TS, Bundred PE. Prevalence, aetiology, and management of heart failure in general practice. *Br J Gen Pract* 1996; 46: 77–79.

82   Eccles M, Freemantle N, Mason J. Group for the North of England ACE-inhibitor Guideline Development. North of England evidence based development project: guideline for angiotensin converting enzyme inhibitors in primary care management of adults with symptomatic heart failure. *BMJ* 1998; 316: 1369–1375.

83   McMurray JJV. Evidence-based medicine in heart failure: towards better treatment. 3. From investigational evidence to daily practice: what are the issues? *Clinician* 1998; 14–20.

84   McMurray J, Davie A. The pharmacoeconomics of ACE inhibitors in chronic heart failure. *Pharmacoeconomics* 1996; 9: 188–197.

85 Doughty RN, Rodgers A, Sharpe N, MacMahon S. Effects of β-blocker therapy on mortality in patients with heart failure. *Eur Heart J* 1997; 18: 560–565.

86 Doughty RN, MacMahon S, Sharpe N. β-blockers in heart failure: promising or proved? *J Am Coll Cardiol* 1997; 23: 814–821.

87 Pfeffer MA, Stevenson LW. β-adrenergic blockers and survival in heart failure. *N Engl J Med* 1996; 334: 1396–1397.

88 Packer M, Bristow MR, Cohn JN *et al.* for the U.S. Carvedilol Heart Failure Study Group. The effect of carvedilol on morbidity and mortality in patients with chronic heart failure. *N Engl J Med* 1996; 334: 1349–1355.

89 Pitt B, Segal R, Martinez FA *et al.* for the ELITE Study Investigators. Randomized trial of losartan versus captopril in patients over 65 with heart failure (Evaluation of Losartan in the Elderly Study, ELITE). *Lancet* 1997; 349: 747–752.

90 Greenberg BM. Medical therapy for patients with aortic insufficiency. *Cardiol Clin* 1991; 9: 255–270.

91 Scognamiglio R, Rahimtoola SH, Fasoli G *et al.* Nifedipine in asymptomatic patients with severe aortic regurgitation and normal left ventricular function. *N Engl J Med* 1994; 331: 689.

92 Greenberg BH, Rahimtoola SH. Long-term vasodilator therapy of chronic aortic insufficiency. *Ann Intern Med* 1980; 93: 440.

93 Le Heuzey JY, Guize L. Cardiac prognosis in hypertensive patients. *Am J Med* 1988; 84 (Suppl. 1B): 65–68.

94 Wolf PA, Abbott RD, Kannel WB. Atrial fibrillation as an independent risk factor for stroke. The Framingham Study. *Stroke* 1991; 22: 983–988.

95 Prystowsky EN, Benson W, Fuster V *et al.* Management of patients with atrial fibrillation. *Circulation* 1996; 93: 1262–1277.

96 Cobbe SM. Using the right drug. A treatment algorithm for atrial fibrillation. *Eur Heart J* 1997; 18 (Suppl. C): C33.

97 The Digitalis in Acute Atrial Fibrillation (DAAF) Trial Group. *Eur Heart J* 1997; 18: 649–654.

98 Jordaens L, Trouerbach J, Calle R *et al.* Conversion of atrial fibrillation to sinus rhythm and rate control by digoxin in comparison to placebo. *Eur Heart J* 1997; 18: 643–648.

99 Cleland JGF, Cowburn PJ, Falk RH. Should all patients with atrial fibrillation receive warfarin? *Eur Heart J* 1996; 17: 674–681.

100 Petersen OP, Boysen G, Godtfredsen J, Andersen ED, Andersen B. Placebo-controlled, randomized trial of warfarin versus aspirin for prevention of thrombo-embolic complications in chronic atrial fibrillation: the Copenhagen AFASAK study. *Lancet* 1989; 1: 175–179.

101 The Boston Area Anticoagulation Trial for Atrial Fibrillation Investigators. The effect of low-dose warfarin on the risk of stroke in patients with non-rheumatic atrial fibrillation. *N Engl J Med* 1990; 323: 1505–1511.

102 Connolly SJ, Laupacis A, Gent M *et al.* Canadian atrial fibrillation anticoagulation (CAFA) study. *J Am Coll Cardiol* 1991; 18: 349–355.

103 Stroke Prevention in Atrial Fibrillation Investigators. Stroke prevention in atrial fibrillation study; final results. *Circulation* 1991; 84: 527–539.

104 Ezekowitz ND, Bridges SL, James KE *et al.* Warfarin in the prevention of stroke associated with non-rheumatic atrial fibrillation. *N Engl J Med* 1992; 327: 1406–1412.

105 European Atrial Fibrillation Study Group. Secondary prevention in non-rheumatic atrial fibrillation after transient ischaemic attack or minor stroke. *Lancet* 1993; 342: 1255–1262.

106   Broderick JP, Phillips SJ, O'Fallon M, Frye RL, Whisnant JP. Relationship of cardiac disease to stroke occurrence, recurrence and mortality. *Stroke* 1992; 23: 1250–1256.

107   Warfarin versus aspirin for prevention of thrombo-embolism in atrial fibrillation. Stroke Prevention in Atrial Fibrillation II Study. *Lancet* 1994; 343: 687–691.

108   Miller VT, Pearce LA, Feinberg WM, Rothrock JF, Anderson DC, Hart RG. Differential effect of aspirin versus warfarin on clinical stroke types in patients with atrial fibrillation. Stroke Prevention in Atrial Fibrillation Investigators. *Neurology* 1996; 46: 238–240.

109   Laupacis A, Boysen G, Connolly S *et al*. Risk factors for stroke and efficacy of antithrombotic therapy in atrial fibrillation: analysis of pooled data from five randomized controlled trials. *Arch Intern Med* 1994; 154: 1449–1457.

110   Zabalgoitia M, Halperin JL, Pearce LA, Blackshear JL, Asinger RW, Hart RG. Transesophageal echocardiographic correlates of clinical risk of thromboembolism in nonvalvular atrial fibrillation. Stroke Prevention in Atrial Fibrillation III Investigators. *J Am Coll Cardiol* 1998; 31: 1622–1626.

111   The Stroke Prevention in Atrial Fibrillation Investigators. Prevention of thromboembolism in atrial fibrillation, II. echocardiographic features of patients at risk. *Ann Intern Med* 1992; 116: 6–12.

112   Petersen P, Kastrup J, Helweg Larsen S, Boysen G, Godtfredsen J. Risk factors for thrombo-embolic complications in chronic atrial fibrillation. The Copenhagen AFASAK Study. *Arch Intern Med* 1990; 150: 819–821.

113   Pearce LA. Predictors of thrombo-embolism in atrial fibrillation: I. Clinical features of patients at risk. *Arch Intern Med* 1992; 116: 1–5.

114   Loh E, St John Sutton M. Anticoagulation and left ventricular dysfunction: friend or foe? *Eur Heart J* 1997; 18: 1039–1041.

115   Benjamin EJ, Plehn JF, D'Agostino RB *et al*. Mitral annular calcification and the risk of stroke in an elderly cohort. *N Engl J Med* 1992; 327: 374–379.

116   Lechat P, Mas JL, Lascault G *et al*. Prevalence of patent foramen ovale in patients with stroke. *N Engl J Med* 1988; 318: 1148–1152.

117   Di Tullio M, Sacco RL, Gopal A, Mohr JP, Homma S. Patent foramen ovale as a risk factor for cryptogenic stroke. *Ann Intern Med* 1992; 117: 461–465.

118   Cabanes L, Mas JLV, Cohen A *et al*. Atrial septal aneurysm and patent foramen ovale as risk factors for cryptogenic stroke in patients less than 55 years of age: a study using transesophageal echocardiography. *Stroke* 1993; 24: 1865–1873.

119   Hylek EM, Skates SJ, Sheenan MA, Singer DE. An analysis of the lowest effective intensity of prophylactic anticoagulation for patients with non-rheumatic atrial fibrillation. *N Engl J Med* 1996; 335: 540–546.

120   Lancaster T, Mant J, Singer DE. Stroke prevention in atrial fibrillation. *BMJ* 1997; 314: 1563–1564.

6: Cerebrovascular Disease

Stroke is a leading cause of death and disability in industrialized nations. In the United States, ≈500 000 people have a new or recurrent stroke and 3 820 000 have survived one [1]. In Europe, age-adjusted mortality from cerebrovascular disease in men ranges from 54 in Switzerland to 606 per 100 000 in the Ukraine, with somewhat lower rates in women (Fig. 6.1).

Hypertension is the most important modifiable risk factor for cerebrovascular disease (Table 6.1). The risk increases with increasing levels of blood pressure in both sexes and at all ages, with [2] or without a previous stroke. The relative risk is approximately fourfold when blood pressures are > 160/95 mmHg, although by the age of 90 the impact of hypertension on stroke decreases (odds ratio of 1) [3]. It is now beyond doubt that treating hypertension dramatically reduces the incidence of stroke. In an overview of 17 treatment trials (involving almost 50 000 patients) antihypertensive treatment was shown to reduce all strokes by 38% and fatal stroke by 40% [4], regardless of age and race (black or white).

STROKE AND TRANSIENT ISCHAEMIC ATTACKS

Distinction between the different categories of cerebrovascular events is imperative in management, be it in the acute situation or in the clinic setting. Cerebrovascular events occurring as a result of cerebrovascular disease can be classified according to duration of the deficit, the pattern of the deficit and its pathogenesis.

Cerebrovascular events can be broadly classified as follows:

Duration of deficit
- Strokes: a neurological deficit lasting > 24 h
- Transient ischaemic attacks (TIA): a neurological deficit lasting < 24 h, but usually lasting minutes or < 1 h

Territory of deficit
- Carotid artery territory
- Vertebrobasilar territory

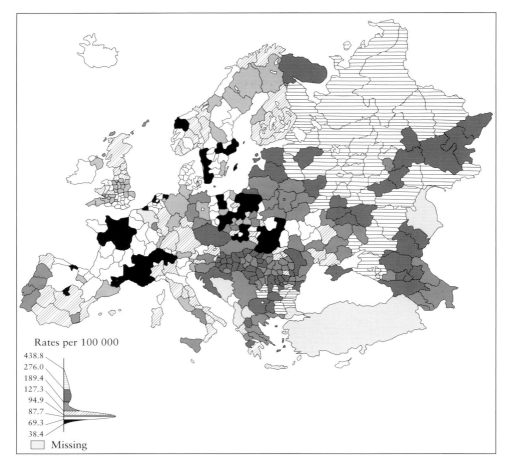

Rates per 100 000

438.8	
276.0	
189.4	
127.3	
94.9	
87.7	
69.3	
38.4	

☐ Missing

Figure 6.1 Age-standardized mortality from cerebrobascular accidents (ICS 430–438) in European regions in 1990–1. Men aged 0–64 years. Reproduced from Sans *et al*. Task Force Report. *Eur Heart J* 1997; 18: 1245. With permission of WB Saunders Co. Ltd, London, UK.

Pathogenesis of deficit

Ischaemic

• In situ thrombosis of an intracranial or neck artery (carotid or vertebral territories)
• Embolism from atheromatous carotid arteries, the aortic arch or the heart
• Reduced cerebral perfusion as a result of the co-existence of hypotension and a critical stenosis in an intracranial artery. Hypotension may be due to antihypertensive treatment *per se*, or to other causes
• Arterial spasm (rare)

Lacunar

• Infarction of territories supplied by small penetrating arteries

Haemorrhagic

• Rupture of Charcot–Bouchard micro-aneurysms

Table 6.1 Risk factors for stroke.

Non-modifiable
Age
Male gender
Black race
Genetic predisposition
Previous stroke or TIA

Modifiable
Hypertension
Cardiac disease
Diabetes
Cigarette smoking
Excessive alcohol intake*
No alcohol intake*
High dose (> 50 μg oestrogen) oral contraceptives†
Illicit drug use

Cocaine	LSD
Heroin	PCP
Amphetamines	'Ts and Blues'
Marijuana	

Aortic arch atheroma‡
Asymptomatic carotid stenosis
Obesity
Lipids?
Physical inactivity?
Migraine?§

*There is a J-shaped association between alcohol intake and risk of stroke [5], with low-to-moderate intake having a protective effect on overall mortality.
†The currently prescribed low-dose oral contraceptives (< 50 μg oestrogen) have been shown not to lead to increased risk of stroke [6].
‡In the Physicians' Health Study, no association was found between migraine and ischaemic stroke after correcting for other risk factors [7]. In young women with migraine, the absolute risk of stroke is very small (rising from 10 to 19 per 100 000).
§Aortic arch atheroma as detected in transoesophageal echocardiography: presence of aortic arch plaque > 4 mm is a marker of high risk for recurrent stroke, MI, peripheral embolism and vascular death.
LSD, lysergic acid diethylamide; PCP, phencyclohexylpiperidine (phencyclidine, angel dust).

The causes of strokes and TIAs are summarized in Fig. 6.2.

DIAGNOSIS

History

A detailed history may reveal symptoms of a stroke or a TIA, which may have gone unreported. A sudden onset and absence of preceding aura or headache are characteristic. Weakness, numbness and paraesthesia are the most common symptoms. The progression of symptoms will define whether the neurological deficit was a stroke (> 24 h) or a TIA (< 24 h). Typically, in both strokes and TIAs, the rate of recovery is slower than the onset of symptoms.

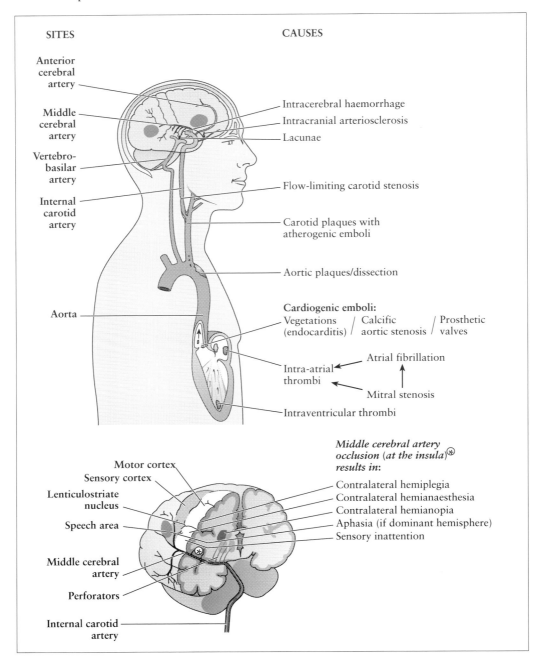

SITES

Anterior cerebral artery

Middle cerebral artery

Vertebro-basilar artery

Internal carotid artery

Aorta

CAUSES

Intracerebral haemorrhage

Intracranial arteriosclerosis

Lacunae

Flow-limiting carotid stenosis

Carotid plaques with atherogenic emboli

Aortic plaques/dissection

Cardiogenic emboli:
Vegetations / Calcific / Prosthetic
(endocarditis) / aortic stenosis / valves

Atrial fibrillation

Intra-atrial thrombi

Mitral stenosis

Intraventricular thrombi

Motor cortex
Sensory cortex
Lenticulostriate nucleus
Speech area

Middle cerebral artery

Perforators

Internal carotid artery

Middle cerebral artery occlusion (at the insula)⊛ results in:

Contralateral hemiplegia
Contralateral hemianaesthesia
Contralateral hemianopia
Aphasia (if dominant hemisphere)
Sensory inattention

Figure 6.2 Causes of stroke and transient ischaemic attacks.

Table 6.2 Distribution of cerebral infarction in patients with a first stroke.

Internal carotid artery*	47%
Lacunar	26%
Vertebrobasilar system†	23%
Unknown	4%

*Either entire (17%) or only part (30%) of the internal carotid territory.
†Includes the posterior cerebral artery territory.
Adapted from data of 515 patients enrolled in the Oxfordshire Community Stroke Project [8].

Scrutiny in the history over the distribution of sensory and motor deficits and the cranial nerves involved may give clues as to the arterial territories affected. The internal carotid territory is the most frequently affected (Table 6.2).

It is extremely unusual for TIAs to cause loss of consciousness unless there is additional pathology, such as cardiac arrhythmia or hypotension. They should be differentiated from focal epilepsy or migraine, which may be preceded by an aura consisting of headache, nausea or vomiting. The diagnosis of a TIA should be reconsidered if there is no focal neurology. Vertebrobasilar TIAs, however, may not produce focal neurology and may manifest as drop attacks or transient global amnesia.

The notion of neck movements causing TIAs through temporary obstruction of a vertebral artery has unfortunately gained popularity. In most cases, TIAs are due to other causes. The history should include detailed questioning regarding concomitant cardiovascular disease and cardiovascular risk factors.

Examination
The clinical examination should be geared towards identifying:
• The arterial territory involved;
• Possible embolic sources;
• Co-existent CHD;
• Other conditions that are unrelated to hypertension but which will influence management.

The patterns of neurological deficit produced by lesions in the different arterial territories are shown in Fig. 6.3. The following general points are worth noting:
• The presence of a carotid bruit during auscultation of the neck is a very unreliable sign of the presence or severity of carotid artery disease [9];
• Cerebrovascular deficits affecting the eye alone have the same implications on management as those affecting cerebral territories;
• Transient monocular blindness (amaurosis fugax) can also be due to retinal ischaemia from other causes other than thromboembolism, e.g. retinal haemorrhage or detachment.

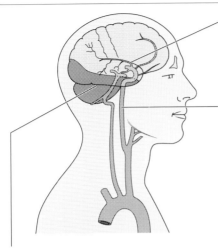

Middle cerebral artery
Aphasia/dysphasia (if dominant hemisphere involved)
Contralateral homonymous hemianopia
Contralateral sensory inattention, hemiplegia
    and/or sensory loss

Internal carotid artery
Deterioration of conscious level
Global aphasia (if dominant hemisphere involved)
Contralateral homonymous hemianopia
Contralateral sensory inattention, hemiplegia/
    sensory loss
Conjugate eye deviation towards side of lesion
Partial Horner's syndrome

Vertebrobasilar artery
Diplopia, visual field loss/binocular blindness
Intermittent memory disturbance
Loss of consciousness
Ataxia, vertigo
Unilateral or bilateral motor or sensory deficit
Deafness, tinnitus
Dysarthria, dysphagia
Nausea, vomiting

Lacunar infarctions

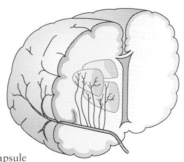

Site of lesion	**Effect**
Anterior limb of internal capsule	Facial weakness + severe dysarthria
Posterior limb of internal capsule	Pure motor hemisyndrome
Postero-lateral thalamus	Pure sensory hemisyndrome
Pons	Clumsy hand-dysarthria syndrome
Pons	Ipsilateral ataxia plus leg weakness
Multiple lacunar infarction	'Marche à petit pas', pseudobulbar palsy and dementia

Figure 6.3 Clinical features of neurological deficit according to arterial territory involved.

Table 6.3 Investigations for patients with acute stroke.

Routine investigations
CT brain, without contrast*
ECG
Chest X-ray
Cervical spine X-rays†
Full blood count
U+Es and glucose
LFTs
Prothrombin time
Partial thromboplastin time

Targeted investigations
CT brain, with contrast
Arterial blood gases (if hypoxia is suspected)
Lumbar puncture (if subarachnoid haemorrhage is suspected and CT is negative)
Electroencephalogram (if seizures suspected)

*If there is no progression in the neurological picture and there are no signs of increased intracranial haemorrhage, computed tomography (CT) of the brain may be performed at a later date.
†If the patient is comatose or has cervical spine pain or tenderness.
LFTs, liver function tests; U+Es, urea and electrolytes.
Adapted from [10].

INVESTIGATION OF ACUTE STROKE

Referral to a centre specialized in the care of stroke is highly recommended [10,11]. The priorities of initial investigations are threefold:
• To differentiate between ischaemic, haemorrhagic and cardioembolic stroke;
• To identify additional pathology which may influence acute management, such as myocardial infarction, cardiac arrhythmias or aortic dissection;
• To identify complications.
    Investigations for patients with stroke or TIAs are shown in Table 6.3.

Computed tomography (CT)

This is the investigation of choice [12] in differentiating between ischaemic and haemorrhagic stroke and in excluding conditions which mimic strokes (Fig. 6.4). The yield of early CT in detecting intracerebral haemorrhage is almost 100% and therefore, the absence of haemorrhage in a patient with neurological deficit can be taken as supporting evidence for an ischaemic stroke. Small subcortical or cortical infarctions as well as posterior fossa infarctions can be missed, even with high-resolution CT. When performed early, the absence of a hypolucent zone does not exclude ischaemic stroke and in this situation, a further CT should be performed in the following days.

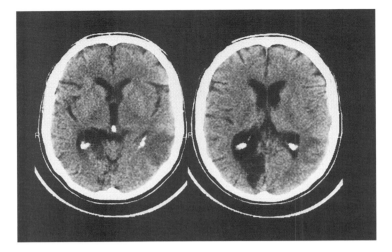

Figure 6.4 Computed tomography scans of patients with a stroke. The region of low attenuation shown in the scan on the left relates to a new stroke involving the watershed areas, which occurred following occlusion of the left carotid artery. On the right is an unenhanced CT scan of the hypertensive patient demonstrating a region of low attenuation involving the occipital lobes. Figure courtesy of Dr Sarah Thorne.

A normal scan or hypodense lesion > 4 weeks after the stroke does not exclude a haemorrhage.

ECG

The fact that the most common cause of death in patients who have survived a stroke is not another stroke, but an MI [13,14] is often overlooked. Evidence of MI and/or cardiac arrhythmias is frequently found in patients with acute ischaemic stroke [15–17]. It is therefore imperative to perform an ECG in all patients with acute or 'old' stroke or TIA. Cardiac monitoring over the 24 h following the stroke may reveal potentially fatal arrhythmias [18,19]. The possibility that an arrhythmia may be the cause of a stroke should also be considered.

Echocardiography

This is unlikely to change the management of acute stroke and should therefore be regarded as an elective investigation. If, however, aortic dissection is suspected, transoesophageal echocardiography should be considered as an alternative to contrast-enhanced CT.

TREATMENT OF ACUTE STROKE

Treatment of acute stroke should ideally take place in a centre specialized in stroke [11]. Airway support and ventilatory measures should be considered if

Table 6.4 Common complications of acute stroke.

Intracranial	Extracranial
Cerebral oedema	Aspiration pneumonia
Hydrocephalus	Hypoventilation
Increased intracranial pressure	Myocardial infarction and ischaemia
Haemorrhagic transformation	Cardiac arrhythmias
Seizures	Neurogenic pulmonary oedema
	Pulmonary embolism
	Urinary tract infections
	Urinary retention
	Pressure sores and ulcers
	Contractures
	Dehydration and malnutrition
	Deep venous thrombosis
	Urinary/faecal incontinence

there is evidence of arterial hypoxaemia, but this issue is contentious. Antipyretics and hypoglycaemic treatment may also be used. Early mobilization and measures to prevent the complications of stroke (Table 6.4) should be implemented and attention should focus on treatment of concurrent infection and other medical conditions. Treatment with prophylactic heparin (5000 U b.d.) for immobilized patients is recommended once a CT scan has shown no evidence of intracranial haemorrhage. Compression stockings are advisable for those who are unable to receive heparin.

Thrombolytic therapy is not currently recommended, unless it is in the context of a clinical trial. Haemodilution, nimodipine, barbiturates, naloxone, glutamate antagonists and amphetamines are not recommended [10]. The role of emergency carotid endarterectomy and angioplasty in acute stroke has not been assessed.

Aspirin

If given early in *non-haemorrhagic* stroke, ideally < 6 h from the onset, aspirin reduces the development of subsequent stroke. It also prevents MI [20], which is likely to occur in up to 2% of stroke patients before they leave hospital.

Unless contra-indicated, *aspirin 300 mg o.d.* should be continued for 2 weeks, then switched to *aspirin 75 mg o.d.* indefinitely.

Antihypertensive treatment in acute stroke

Blood pressure rises in response to a stroke in previously non-hypertensive and hypertensive individuals. Evidence relating to treatment thresholds for antihypertensive therapy is scarce, but the consensus is that blood pressure treatment in the acute phase of a stroke should not be commenced unless the systolic pressure is > 200 mmHg or the calculated mean blood pressure [systolic blood + (2 × diastolic)/3] is > 130 mmHg [10,21,22]. It should be noted that responses to antihypertensive drugs may be exaggerated in the acute phase of a stroke [21,23]. The decision about whether to treat or not should be made over a period of hours. There is evidence to suggest that antihypertensive treatment can jeopardize the zone of cerebral infarction by inducing further ischaemia. A smooth reduction in blood pressure over a period of hours is preferable to sudden reductions, which may compromise 'watershed' areas of the brain. Intravenous therapy should be considered if there is accompanying haemorrhagic transformation, heart failure, aortic dissection, acute renal failure or MI.

Little is known about the effects on clinical outcome of the different antihypertensive drugs in the acute phase of a stroke. Vasodilators, such as hydralazine [24] and sodium nitroprusside [25], may increase intracranial pressure and may therefore encourage cerebral haemorrhage. Calcium antagonists may reduce blood flow in peri-infarct ischaemic areas through a 'steal' phenomenon, and may also raise intracranial pressure and produce profound hypotension [10]. Although ACE inhibitors do not appear to exert these effects, they may cause profound hypotension in acute stroke and are therefore unsuitable in this situation. Labetalol, which combines α- and β-blocking properties, does not increase intracranial pressure and its blood pressure lowering effects are eminently manageable.

SECONDARY PREVENTION OF CEREBROVASCULAR DISEASE

The most important threat to life in patients who have survived a stroke is not another stroke, but an MI. Likewise, patients with asymptomatic carotid stenosis more commonly die from cardiac events than from stroke [13,14]. In carotid stenosis, the risk of a stroke rises with the degree of stenosis [26] approaching a maximum at 75–90% [27]. Once a TIA has occurred, the risk of stroke increases markedly [13,26], being highest in the ensuing weeks or months [28]. On average, the risk of a future stroke and/or death is about 10% per annum. The risk of a first stroke rises with increasing age, the presence of CHD and excessive alcohol consumption (Table 6.5).

It is clear from the above that management of patients with cerebrovascular disease involves management of their CHD risk. This involves a joint approach to risk factor management.

Non-pharmacological intervention
This is dealt with in Chapter 11 and non-pharmacological treatment is summarized in Table 6.6.

Table 6.5 Age-adjusted incidence (per 1000/year) of a first stroke in men, according to alcohol consumption and presence of pre-existing coronary heart disease.

Myocardial infarction*	4.2
Heavy alcohol consumption†	3.3
Angina/myocardial ischaemia	2.6
None/occasional/moderate alcohol intake	1.8
Light alcohol intake	1.3

*Diagnosis of myocardial infarction made on the basis of clinical history and Rose chest pain questionnaire and ECG.
†Alcohol intake in drinks/week: never or occasional = 1; light = 1–20; moderate = 21–42; heavy > 42.
Adapted from [29].

Table 6.6 Lifestyle modifications for hypertensive patients with cerebrovascular disease.*

- Stop smoking
- Lose weight to keep BMI between 20 and 25 kg m^{-2}. Aim to lose 0.5–1 kg week^{-1} (not more) by avoiding fatty foods, sugar and alcohol. Crash diets do not help in the long term
- Limit alcohol intake to 28 units per week in men and to 21 units per week in women, without bingeing
- Walk briskly for ~45 min per day on most days of the week
- Keep a good diet for reducing coronary risk:
  Avoid processed foods
  Keep daily salt (sodium chloride) intake < 6 g day^{-1} by†:
     Avoiding processed foods and other salty foods
     Avoiding adding salt at the table
  Keep a low daily total and saturated fat intake
  Eat fresh fruit and vegetables with every meal
  Eat foods containing soluble fibre at least once a day
  Eat fish at least three times a week

*Advice on all points mentioned is supported by data from observational studies rather than randomized prospective studies.
†Whether salt intake should be reduced in normotensive patients is a contentious issue which has not been adequately addressed by any study.
BMI, body mass index.

Pharmacological intervention

A summary of the pharmacological interventions available for the joint risk factor management is shown in Table 6.7.

Aspirin. Patients who have had a stroke or TIA should be taking 75 mg o.d. indefinitely. Dipyridamole was shown not to be of benefit in a large meta-analysis [20], but some evidence suggests that the modified-release preparation may confer some benefit [31]. At present, *slow-release dipyridamole 200 mg b.d.* should be reserved as an alternative in patients who are intolerant of aspirin [i.e. those with a history of hypersensitivity (asthma, angio-oedema, urticaria, rhinitis) or those at high risk of bleeding (*active* peptic

Table 6.7 Drug treatment for hypertensive patients who have suffered a stroke or a transient ischaemic attack (TIA).

Aspirin*	300 mg o.d. for 2 weeks following the stroke or TIA, then switching to 75 mg o.d. indefinitely†
Antihypertensive therapy	Thiazides or β-blockers to keep blood pressure < 130/85 mmHg
Statins	Simvastatin or pravastatin indefinitely, to keep LDL-cholesterol < 3.0 mmol l^{-1}
Anticoagulant therapy	Warfarin, indefinitely, if embolic predisposition‡

*Modified-release dypiridamole should be reserved for patients who have had a stroke or a TIA who cannot tolerate aspirin.
†Switching to the lower dose is recommended to minimize the risks of gastrointestinal haemorrhage [30].
‡See p. 77.
BMI, body mass index; LDL-cholesterol, low-density lipoprotein cholesterol.

ulceration and *not* just a history of ulcers, recent injury or bleeding diathesis)]. The evidence for a superior benefit of combined aspirin and dipyridamole is conflicting [31–33].

Anticoagulant therapy. This is currently indicated only in patients who have had a stroke or a TIA and in whom a cardiac condition predisposing to embolism has been identified (p. 77). The target international normalized ratio (INR) for non-rheumatic AF in patients who have had a previous stroke or TIA is 2.0–3.9 (p. 78).

Antihypertensive treatment. Thiazides and β-blockers have confidently been shown to prevent strokes. Because the large trials of antihypertensive treatment have not incorporated cerebral imaging techniques, no distinction has been made between the different types of strokes nor indeed, their possibly different responses to antihypertensive treatment. Some studies do suggest a different treatment response [34]. Such trials have not incorporated measures of 'severity' of stroke and it is therefore impossible to ascertain whether different types of treatment have variable effects on cerebral infarct size. It should be noted that antihypertensive treatment also prevents TIAs [35].

African–Caribbean patients are particularly prone to the complications of hypertension [36,37]. We recommend therefore that in black people who have had a stroke, a goal of < 135/85 mmHg is adopted in antihypertensive management.

Statins. Hypercholesterolaemia does not emerge as a risk factor for stroke [29,38–40]. However, in a recent meta-analysis (16 trials, ≈ 29 000 patients, average follow-up 3.3 years) [41] lipid-lowering therapy with statins was associated with a 29% reduction in risk of stroke. In another meta-analysis of randomized trials (28 trials, $\approx$ 49 000 in intervention group and 56 000 in the control group [42]), the risk ratio for non-fatal and fatal stroke with statins was 0.76, which was highly significant. Similar findings have emerged from other subanalyses of patients with stroke [41,43]. In contrast to statins, the risk ratios for fibrates, resins and dietary modification were all close to 1.0, indicating that these measures confer no benefit with respect to stroke incidence.

There is insufficient evidence to justify the use of statins in the primary prevention of stroke. However, the evidence of benefits in patients with stroke is sufficiently compelling [44–46] to justify the same approach as in patients with CHD (i.e. to keep total cholesterol $\leq$ 5.0 mmol l^{-1} and LDL-cholesterol < 3.0 mmol l^{-1}) (p. 116).

References

1 American Heart Association. *Heart and Stroke Facts: 1996 Statistical Supplement*. Dallas, TX, 1995.
2 Rodgers A, McMahon S, Gamble G *et al*. Blood pressure and risk of stroke in patients with cerebrovascular disease. *BMJ* 1996; 313: 147.
3 Whisnant JP. Effectiveness versus efficacy of treatment of hypertension for stroke prevention. *Neurology* 1996; 46: 301–307.
4 McMahon S, Rodgers A. The epidemiological association between blood pressure and stroke: implications for primary and secondary prevention. *Hypertens Res* 1994; 17 (Suppl. 1): S23–S32.
5 Camargo CA Jr. Moderate alcohol consumption and stroke: the epidemiologic evidence. *Stroke* 1989; 269: 1611–1626.
6 Petitti DB, Sidney S, Bernstein A, Wolf S, Quesenberry C, Ziel HK. Stroke in users of low-dose oral contraceptives. *N Engl J Med* 1996; 335: 8–15.
7 Buring JE, Hebert P, Romero J *et al*. Migraine and subsequent risk of stroke in the Physicians Health Study. *Arch Neurol* 1995; 52: 129–134.
8 Warlow CP. Cerebrovascular disease. In: Weatherall D, Ledingham J, Warrel D, eds. *Oxford Textbook of Medicine*, Vol. 2. Oxford: Oxford University Press, 1989: 21.155–21.181.
9 Davies KN, Humphrey PRD. Do carotid bruits predict disease of the internal carotid artery? *Postgrad Med J* 1994; 70: 433–435.
10 Adams HP, Brott TG, Crowell RM *et al*. Guidelines for the management of patients with acute ischemic stroke. *Circulation* 1994; 90 (3): 1588–1601.
11 Langhorne P, Williams BO, Gilchrist W, Howle K. Do stroke units save lives? *Lancet* 1993; 342: 395–398.
12 Bamford J. Clinical examination in diagnosis and subclassification of stroke. *Lancet* 1992; 339: 400–402.
13 Norris JW, Zhu CZ, Bornstein NM, Chambers BR. Vascular risks of asymptomatic carotid stenosis. *Stroke* 1991; 22: 1485–1490.
14 Hennerici M, Hülsbömer H-B, Hefter H, Lammerts D, Rautenberg W. Natural history of asymptomatic extracranial arterial disease. Results of a long-term prospective study. *Brain* 1987; 110: 777–791.

15 Bamford J, Dennis M, Sandercock P, Burn J, Warlow C. The frequency, causes and timing of death within 30 days of a first stroke. The Oxfordshire Community Stroke Project. *J Neurol Neurosurg Psychiat* 1990; 53: 824–829.

16 Broderick JP, Phillips SJ, O'Fallon M, Frye RL, Whisnant JP. Relationship of cardiac disease to stroke occurrence, recurrence and mortality. *Stroke* 1992; 23: 1250–1256.

17 Vingerhoets F, Bogousslavsky J, Regli F, Van Melle G. Atrial fibrillation after acute stroke. *Stroke* 1993; 24: 26–30.

18 Oppenheimer SM, Hachinski VC. The cardiac consequences of stroke. *Neurol Clin N Am* 1992; 10: 167–176.

19 DiPasquale G, Urbinati S, Pinelli G. Cardiac arrhythmias following acute brain injuries. In: DiPasquale G, Pinelli G, eds. *Heart–Brain Interactions*. Berlin: Springer-Verlag, 1992: 212–274.

20 Antiplatelet Trialist's Collaboration. Collaborative overview of randomised trials of antiplatelet treatment. Part I. Prevention of death, myocardial infarction and stroke by prolonged antiplatelet therapy in various categories of patients. *BMJ* 1994; 308: 81–106.

21 American Heart Association Emergency Cardiac Care Committee and Sub-committees. Guidelines for cardiopulmonary resuscitation and emergency cardiac care. *JAMA* 1992; 268: 2242–2250.

22 Powers WJ. Acute hypertension after stroke. *Neurology* 1993; 43: 461–467.

23 Britton M, de Faire U, Helmers C. Hazards of therapy for excessive hypertension in acute stroke. *Acta Med Scand* 1980; 207: 253–257.

24 Overgaard J, Skinhøj E. Dihydralazine induces marked cerebral vasodilation in man. *Eur J Clin Invest* 1975; 17: 214–217.

25 Turner JM, Powell D, Gibson RM, McDowall DG. Intracranial pressure changes in neurosurgical patients during hypotension induced with sodium nitroprusside or trimetaphan. *Br J Anaesthesiol* 1977; 49: 419–420.

26 Mackey AE, Abrahamowicz M, Langlois Y *et al*. Outcome of asymptomatic patients with carotid disease. *Neurology* 1997; 48: 896–903.

27 Norris JW, Zhu CZ. Stroke risk and critical carotid stenosis. *J Neurol Neurosurg Psychiat* 1990; 53: 235–237.

28 Warlow CP, Dennis MS, van Gijn J *et al*. *Stroke: A Practical Guide to Management*. Oxford: Blackwell Science, 1996: 545–597.

29 Shaper AG, Phillips AN, Podock SJ, Walker M, McFarlane PW. Risk factors for stroke in middle aged British men. *BMJ* 1991; 302: 1111–1115.

30 Which prophylactic aspirin? *Drug Ther Bull* 1997; 35: 7–8.

31 Diener HC, Cunha L, Forbes C, Sivenius J, Smets P, Lowenthal A. European Stroke Prevention Study 2. Dipyridamole and acetylsalicylic acid in the secondary prevention of stroke. *J Neurol Sci* 1996; 143: 1–13.

32 American-Canadian Co-operative Study Group. Persantin aspirin trial in cerebral ischemia. Part II. Endpoint results. *Stroke* 1983; 16: 406–415.

33 Bousser MG, Eschwege E, Hagenah M *et al*. 'AICLA' controlled trial of aspirin and dipyridamole in the secondary prevention of athero-thrombotic cerebral ischemia. *Stroke* 1983; 14: 5–14.

34 Spence JD. Antihypertensive drugs and prevention of atherosclerotic stroke. *Stroke* 1986; 17: 808–810.

35 SHEP Cooperative Research Group. Prevention of stroke by antihypertensive drug treatment in older persons with isolated systolic hypertension: final results of the Systolic Hypertension in the Elderly Program (SHEP). *JAMA* 1991; 265: 3255–3264.

36 Cruickshank JK. National history of blood pressure in black populations. In: Cruickshank J, Beevers D, eds. *Ethnic Factors in Health and Disease*, Vol. 13D. London: Butterworth Heinemann, 1989: 268–279.

37 Wild S, McKeigue P, Cross-sectional analysis of mortality by country of birth in England and E Wales, 1970–92. *BMJ* 1997; 31: 705–710.

38 Neaton JD, Kullen LH, Wentworth D, Borhani NO. Total and cardiovascular mortality in relation to cigarette smoking, serum cholesterol concentration and diastolic blood pressure among black and white males followed up for five years. *Am Heart J* 1984; 108: 759–769.

39 Donnan GA, McNeil JJ, Adena MA, Doyle AF, O'Malley HM, Neill GC. Smoking as a risk factor for cerebral ischaemia. *Lancet* 1989; ii: 643–647.

40 Fuller JH, Shipley MJ, Rose G, Jarrett RJ, Keen H. Mortality from coronary heart disease and stroke in relation to degree of glycaemia: the Whitehall Study. *BMJ* 1983; 287: 867–870.

41 Hebert PR, Gaziano JM, Chan KS, Hennekens CH. Cholesterol lowering with statin drugs, risk of stroke, and total mortality: an overview of randomized trials. *JAMA* 1997; 278: 313–321.

42 Bucher HC, Griffith LE, Guyatt GH. Effect of HMG CoA reductase inhibitors on stroke: a meta-analysis of randomised, controlled trials. *Ann Intern Med* 1998; 128: 89–95.

43 Crouse JR III, Byington RP, Hoen HM, Furberg CD. Reductase inhibitor monotherapy and stroke prevention. *Arch Intern Med* 1997; 157: 1305–1310.

44 Summary of the Second Report of the National Cholesterol Education Program (NECP) Expert Panel on Detection Evaluation, Treatment of High Blood Cholesterol in Adults (Adult Treatment Panel II). *JAMA* 1993; 269: 3015–3023.

45 Feinberg WM, Albers GW, Barnett HJM *et al*. Guidelines for the management of transient ischemic attacks. *Circulation* 1994; 6: 2950–2965.

46 LaRosa JC, Hunninghake D, Bush D *et al*. The cholesterol facts: a summary of the evidence relating dietary fats, serum cholesterol, and coronary heart disease. A joint statement by the American Heart Association and the National Heart, Lung and Blood Institute: the Task Force on Cholesterol Issues, American Heart Association. *Circulation* 1990; 81: 1721–1733.

7: Diabetes Mellitus and Insulin Resistance

Hypertension, diabetes and coronary heart disease (CHD) occur so frequently together that the clinician should regard them as part of a wider disorder, or syndrome. We have no appropriate name for this constellation of diseases, nor have we determined a common underlying cause. What is clear, however, is that clinicians who deal with patients who have any one of these mutually supporting conditions should be familiar with the management of all of them.

HYPERTENSION AND TYPE II DIABETES MELLITUS

Hypertension is commonly associated with diabetes mellitus [1–3]. About 80% of diabetic patients aged 60 years have a blood pressure greater than 140/90 mmHg. In patients with diabetes, hypertension increases mortality by about 1.8-fold [4]. Almost half of patients with newly diagnosed type II diabetes mellitus are hypertensive [5,6] and the excess of hypertension in diabetics compared to non-diabetics is apparent at all ages [7], being more pronounced in women than in men [8].

In managing patients with hypertension and diabetes, we should also consider that both of these conditions are frequently associated with CHD and cerebrovascular disease [9,10]. Type II diabetes mellitus is associated with approximately a twofold increase in CHD in men and a fourfold increase in women [11–13]. In diabetic patients, cardiovascular mortality is also higher (Table 7.1) at all levels of blood pressure [14]. Likewise, the severity of myocardial disease is much increased when hypertension and diabetes co-exist [15]. In addition, hypertension accelerates all the vascular complications associated with diabetes, including those of the retinal, renal, cardiac and the peripheral vasculature [16–19].

It has only recently been shown that the risk factors for CHD in patients with type II diabetes mellitus are similar to those in non-diabetic individuals. These include elevated blood pressures, high low-density lipoprotein (LDL)-cholesterol, low high-density lipoprotein (HDL)-cholesterol, hyperglycaemia and smoking [20].

Table 7.1 Excess of cardiovascular and cerebrovascular disease in diabetic subjects.

Cardiovascular system
↑ Incidence of MI [10,21,22,29]
↑ Infarct size [23] and infarct extension [24]
↑ Re-infarction [10]
↑ Acute complications of MI [10]
↑ Heart failure after MI [10,24]
↑ Mortality after MI, short and long term [25,26]
↑ Angina, silent and symptomatic [10]
↑ Angiographic coronary heart disease [27]
↑ Restenosis after coronary angioplasty [10]
↑ Incidence of systolic/diastolic and isolated systolic hypertension
↑ Left ventricular hypertrophy? [28]
↑ Microangiopathy (gangrene etc.)

Cerebrovascular disease
↑ Mortality [29]

Kidney
↑ Micro-albuminuria
↑ Renal artery stenosis, unilateral and bilateral [30]
↑ Renovascular hypertension
↑ Nephrotic syndrome

Eyes
Macular oedema
Retinopathy

Peripheral vasculature
↑ Peripheral vascular disease [21,29]

Autonomic nervous system
Peripheral somatic neuropathy
Cardiac autonomic dysfunction [31,32]

DIAGNOSIS OF DIABETES

Screening for diabetes should routinely be carried out in all hypertensive patients and also, in all patients with cardiac, peripheral vascular, retino-vascular or cerebrovascular disease, i.e. all those with suspected or confirmed atherosclerosis. Routine screening for diabetes should also be carried out in patients with dyslipidaemia, particularly those from southern Asia.

The screening investigation of hypertensive patients should include measurement of fasting glucose and of glycosylated haemoglobin (Hb A_{1C}). If fasting glucose levels are between 5.0 and 7.0 mmol l^{-1} or the Hb A_{1C} is elevated, a 75-g oral glucose tolerance test (OGTT) should be performed. The diagnostic thresholds are as follows:

Diabetes certain (on repeated testing)
Fasting plasma glucose > 7.0 mmol l^{-1}
2-h OGTT plasma glucose > 11.1 mmol l^{-1}

Highly suggestive of diabetes
Random plasma glucose > 8.9 mmol l^{-1}

Routine follow-up of diabetic patients is summarized in Table 7.2. Close supervision is required for patients with signs of target-organ damage, those with concomitant cardiovascular disease or other cardiovascular risk factors and those with micro-albuminuria [33,34].

Table 7.2 Routine follow-up of diabetic patients.

Clinical assessment
Blood pressure twice a year, checking lying/standing blood pressure in patients with postural symptoms
Fundoscopy at least annually

Investigations
Lipids: fasting cholesterol, triglycerides and HDL-cholesterol, at least twice a year
Fasting glucose, haemoglobin A_{1C} or fructosamine at least twice a year
Urinalysis, at least annually
  Micro-albuminuria*†: check using a morning urine specimen and a dipstick‡. If the dipstick result is positive, a 24-h urine collection should be obtained [35,36]. If there is persistent micro-albuminuria, optimize antihypertensive therapy and consider ACE inhibitors.

*In insulin-dependent diabetes mellitus (IDDM), micro-albuminuria is an excellent predictor of nephropathy [37,38] and retinopathy [39]. It is also a strong predictor of early death in non-insulin-dependent diabetes mellitus (NIDDM) [40–42].
†Screening for micro-albuminuria should be performed in all patients with IDDM > 12 years and all NIDDM patients from the time of diagnosis until the age of 70 [43]. Micro-albuminuria should be suspected if urine albumin concentration is > 20 mg l^{-1} or urine albumin/creatinine ratio is > 2.5 mg mmol^{-1}. In management, the practicable definitions of micro- and macro-albuminuria are as follows: *Micro-albuminuria*: if two out of three urine collections over a period of 3 months yield an albumin excretion rate (AER) between 30 and 300 mg/24 h (20–200 µg min^{-1}, or 300 mg l^{-1}); *Macro-albuminuria*: if two out of three urine collections yield an AER > 300 mg/24 h (> 200 µg min^{-1}, or > 300 mg l^{-1}).
‡The Micral-Test II (Boehringer Mannheim, Germany) and the Nycocard U-Albumin test (Nycomed Pharma AS, Oslo, Norway) provide simple and rapid (albeit relatively costly) methods for the bedside or clinic measurement of urinary albumin excretion. Some authorities recommend measurement of AER every 3–6 months in diabetic patients, but this may not lead to changes in management in patients who are already receiving treatment aimed at reducing AER.

ANTIHYPERTENSIVE TREATMENT IN DIABETIC PATIENTS

Before completion of the HOT study, evidence suggested that hypertension should be treated more aggressively in diabetic patients [44,45]. The HOT study allowed comparison of outcomes between three randomized blood pressure target groups (≤ 90, 85 or 80 mmHg) and it showed no difference in the risk of developing cardiovascular disease between adjacent target groups in non-diabetic patients [46]. In diabetic patients, however, lowering diastolic blood pressure < 80 mmHg resulted in significant reductions in cardiovascular events. Similarly, in the UKPDS 38, lowering blood pressure to 144/82 mmHg rather than to 154/87 mmHg was associated with significantly lower risks of major macrovascular events and microvascular disease outcomes [47]. This is consistent with the observed benefits of more aggressive blood pressure lowering in normotensive diabetic subjects with or without renal disease.

> On the basis of the above, the WHO-ISH recommend that in diabetic hypertensive patients, the treatment goal should be < 130/85 mmHg [48].

Thiazides and β-blockers

There is heated debate as to whether the presence of diabetes should constitute an automatic indication for the use of the newer antihypertensive agents. On one hand, thiazides and β-blockers *at high doses* are known to induce insulin resistance and hyperinsulinaemia [49,50]. On the other hand, there is little evidence from large trials that the adverse effects of thiazides and β-blockers on glucose metabolism translate to an increase in the incidence of diabetes or, indeed, that low-dose diuretics produce significant, untoward metabolic effects [51]. In this respect it should be noted that diabetic patients who are treated with thiazide diuretics and β-blockers experience a similar or greater reductions in total cardiovascular events compared to non-diabetics [52].

Although β-blockers may mask the symptoms of hypoglycaemia in young diabetics, this is seldom a problem in type II diabetics.

Angiotensin-converting enzyme (ACE) inhibitors

Nephropathy develops in up to 40% of diabetic individuals and is present in 3% of patients with non-insulin-dependent diabetes mellitus (NIDDM) at the time of diagnosis [53]. In both insulin-dependent diabetes mellitus (IDDM) and NIDDM, proteinuria is associated with an increased risk of developing chronic renal failure. Micro-albuminuria occurs early in the course of diabetes and has been shown to predict the development of nephropathy in patients with IDDM and, to a lesser extent, in patients with NIDDM [54]. In patients with IDDM, micro-albuminuria is associated with elevated blood pressure, dyslipidaemia, insulin resistance and increased cardiovascular morbidity and mortality.

Although the UKPDS 39 has shown that the benefits of ACE inhibitors and β-blockers were similar in terms of macrovascular and microvascular outcomes in patients with type II diabetes [47], there is a wealth of evidence in favour of using ACE inhibitors to retard the progression of renal disease in diabetic patients with proteinuria. ACE inhibitors reduce micro-albuminuria and prevent deterioration in renal function in diabetic [55–58] and non-diabetic [59–61] hypertensive patients. The risk of death, the need for dialysis and for renal transplantation in patients with NIDDM can be reduced by one-half using captopril [1]. In addition, ACE inhibitors delay the progression of diabetic renal disease and lessen the increases in micro-albuminuria in diabetic patients, both hypertensive and normotensive [62,63]. The addition of a thiazide diuretic does not adversely affect micro-albuminuria. The renal effects appear to be characteristic of most ACE inhibitors and not particular drugs, i.e. it is a 'class effect'.

α-Blockers

As well as being effective antihypertensive agents, α-blockers improve the lipid profile. Doxazosin reduces total and LDL-cholesterol and triglycerides and increases HDL-cholesterol in non-diabetic [64,65] and diabetic [66] individuals. Compared to thiazides and β-blockers, both prazosin [67] and doxazosin [65] are associated with a better lipid profile after 1 year of treatment. Small, non-controlled studies have linked the beneficial lipid effects of α-blockers to their ability to reduce insulin levels and to improve insulin sensitivity [68]. It should be noted, however, that further studies are needed to determine whether such apparent improvements in glucose metabolism translate to a clinically significant effect.

LIPID LOWERING TREATMENT IN DIABETES

No randomized trials of lipid lowering treatment have focused specifically on diabetic hypertensive patients. It is noteworthy, however, that in the 4S study (simvastatin in the secondary prevention of CHD) [69], treatment with simvastatin led to greater reductions in major coronary events in diabetics than in non-diabetics. This is discussed in Chapter 8.

THE METABOLIC OR 'INSULIN RESISTANCE' SYNDROME

Not only is hypertension commonly found in diabetic patients, but it is also frequently found in association with other metabolic risk factors for CHD. In recognition of the common association of diabetes mellitus, hypertension, obesity, low plasma HDL-cholesterol and hypertriglyceridaemia, the concept of a metabolic syndrome of cardiovascular risk, the so-called

Table 7.3 Proposed components of a metabolic syndrome of cardiovascular risk.

Clinically relevant
Non-insulin dependent diabetes mellitus
↑ Blood pressure
↑ Serum uric acid
↑ Plasma triglycerides
↑ Plasma LDL-cholesterol
↓ Plasma HDL and HDL$_2$-cholesterol
↓ Glucose tolerance
↑ Proportion of central (android) fat

Of research interest
↓ Insulin sensitivity
↑ Plasma insulin
↑ Plasma insulin propeptides
↑ Plasma leptin
↑ Proportion of LDL-cholesterol subtype B
↑ Non-sterified fatty acid flux
↑ Plasminogen activator inhibitor-1
↓ Arterial wall compliance
↓ Arterial blood flow

insulin resistance syndrome, has emerged. Since its description [70], many components have been added [71–75] (Table 7.3). Yet we have no threshold of measurement above or below which to diagnose it [76]. Moreover, although the syndrome appears to predict the development of NIDDM, no studies have explored whether the syndrome itself predicts the development of CHD. Thus, the insulin resistance syndrome should not be regarded as a clinical entity to be diagnosed or treated in individual patients, despite proposed strategies [73]. As an epidemiological entity, however, the concept of the insulin resistance 'syndrome' is helpful in clinical management, insofar as it alerts the clinician to consider the various components of metabolism in patients with hypertension, diabetes and both coronary and cerebrovascular disease.

References

1   Weidmann P. Hypertension and diabetes. In: Kaplan N, ed. *Metabolic Aspects of Hypertension*. London: Science Press, 1994: 2.1–2.23.

2   Weidmann P, Boehlen LM, de Courten M. Pathogenesis and treatment of hypertension associated with diabetes mellitus. *Am Heart J* 1993; 125: 1498–1513.

3   Simonsson DC. Etiology and prevalence of hypertension in diabetic patients. *Diabetes Care* 1988; 11: 821–827.

4   Morrish NJ, Stevens LK, Head J *et al.* A prospective study of mortality among middle-aged diabetic patients (the London cohort of the WHO Multinational Study of Vascular Disease in Diabetics.) II. Associated risk factors. *Diabetologia* 1990; 33: 542–548.

5 Turner RC, Mann J, Oakes S *et al.* United Kingdom Prospective Diabetes Study, a multicenter study. *Hypertension* 1985; 7 (Suppl. II): 8–13.

6 Tarnow L, Rossing P, Gall M *et al.* Prevalence of arterial hypertension in diabetic patients after the JNC-V. *Diabetes Care* 1994; 17: 1247–1251.

7 Krolewski AS, Warram JH, Cupples A, Gorman CK, Szabo AJ, Christlieb AR. Hypertension, orthostatic hypotension and the microvascular complications of diabetes. *J Chron Dis* 1985; 38: 319–326.

8 Ferrannini E, Natali A. Hypertension, insulin resistance and diabetes. In: Swales J, ed. *Textbook of Hypertension*. Oxford: Blackwell Scientific Publications, 1994: 785–797.

9 Jarrett RJ. The epidemiology of coronary heart disease and related factors in the context of diabetes mellitus and impaired glucose tolerance. In: Jarrett RJ, ed. *Diabetes and Heart Disease*. Amsterdam: Elsevier, 1984: 1–24.

10 Pyörälä K, Laakso M, Uusitupa M. Diabetes and atherosclerosis: an epidemiologic view. *Diabetes Metab Rev* 1987; 3: 463–524.

11 Panzram G. Mortality and survival in type 2 (non-insulin-dependent) diabetes mellitus. *Diabetologia* 1987; 30: 123–131.

12 Pan W-H, Cedres LB, Liu K *et al.* Relationship of clinical diabetes and asymptomatic hyperglycemia to risk of coronary heart disease mortality in men and women. *Am J Epidemiol* 1986; 123: 504–516.

13 Fontbonne A, Charles MA, Thibult N *et al.* Hyperinsulinaemia as a predictor of coronary heart disease mortality in a healthy population: the Paris Prospective Study, 15-year follow-up. *Diabetologia* 1991; 34: 356–361.

14 Stamler J, Vaccaro O, Neaton JD, Wentworth D. Diabetes, other risk factors, and 12-yr cardiovascular mortality for men screened in the multiple risk factor intervention trial. *Diabetes Care* 1993; 16: 434–444.

15 Giles TD, Sander GE. Myocardial disease in hypertensive-diabetic patients. *Am J Med* 1989; 87 (Suppl. 6A): 235–285.

16 Kannel WB, McGee DL. Diabetes and cardiovascular risk factors: The Framingham study. *Circulation* 1979; 59: 8–13.

17 Fuller JH, Shipley MJ, Rose G, Jarrett RJ, Keen H. Mortality from coronary heart disease and stroke in relation to degree of glycaemia: the Whitehall Study. *BMJ* 1983; 287: 867–870.

18 Van Hoeven K, Factor S. A comparison of the pathological spectrum of hypertensive, diabetic, and hypertensive-diabetic heart disease. *Circulation* 1990; 82: 848–855.

19 Klein R, Klein BEK, Moss SE *et al.* Is blood pressure a predictor of the incidence or progression of diabetic retinopathy? *Arch Intern Med* 1989; 149: 2427–2432.

20 Turner RC, Neil HAW, Stratton IM *et al.* Risk factors for coronary artery disease in non-insulin dependent diabetes mellitus: United Kingdom prospective diabetes study (UKPDS: 23). *BMJ* 1998; 316: 823–828.

21 Waller BF, Palumbo PJ, Lie JT, Roberts WC. Status of the coronary arteries at necropsy in diabetes mellitus with onset after age 30 years: analysis of 229 diabetic patients with and without clinical evidence of coronary heart disease and comparison of 183 control subjects. *Am J Med* 1980; 69: 498–506.

22 Woods KL, Samanta A, Burden AC. Diabetes mellitus as a risk factor for acute myocardial infarction in Asians and Europeans. *Br Heart J* 1989; 62: 118–122.

23 Rennert G, Saltz-Rennerts H, Wanderman K, Weitzman S. Size of acute myocardial infarct in patients with diabetes mellitus. *Am J Cardiol* 1985; 55: 1629–1630.

24 Stone PH, Muller JE, Hartwell T *et al.* The effect of diabetes mellitus on prognosis and serial left ventricular function after acute myocardial infarction: Contribution of

both coronary disease and diastolic left ventricular dysfunction to adverse prognosis. *J Am Coll Cardiol* 1989; 14: 49–57.

25 Smith JW, Marcus FI, Serokman R, Group with the Multicenter Post-infarction Research. Prognosis of patients with diabetes mellitus after acute myocardial infarction. *Am J Cardiol* 1984; 54: 718–721.

26 Abbott RD, Donahue RP, Kannel WB, Wilson PW. The impact of diabetes on survival following myocardial infarction in men vs women, The Framingham Study. *JAMA* 1988; 260: 3456–3460.

27 Vigorita VJ, Moore GW, Hutchins GM. Absence of correlation between coronary arterial atherosclerosis and severity or duration of diabetes mellitus of adult onset. *Am J Cardiol* 1980; 46: 535–542.

28 Hara-Nakamura N, Kohara K, Suminoto T, Lin M, Hiwada K. Glucose intolerance exaggerates left ventricular hypertrophy and dysfunction in essential hypertension. *Am J Hypertens* 1994; 7: 1110–1114.

29 Kannel WB, McGree DL. Diabetes and glucose tolerance as risk factors for cardiovascular disease. *Diabetes Care* 1979; 2: 120–126.

30 Sawicki PT, Kaiser S, Heinemann L, Frenzel H, Berger M. Prevalence of renal artery stenosis in diabetes mellitus — an autopsy study. *J Int Med* 1991; 229: 489–492.

31 Roy THM, Peterson HR, Snider HL *et al.* Autonomic influence on cardiovascular performance in diabetic patients. *Am J Med* 1989; 87: 382–388.

32 Weise F, Heydenreich F, Gehrig W, Runge U. Heart rate variability in diabetic patients during orthostatic load — a spectral analytic approach. *Klin Wochenschr* 1990; 68: 26.

33 Marré M, Chatellier G, Leblanc H *et al.* Prevention of diabetic nephropathy with enalapril in normotensive diabetics with microalbuminuria. *BMJ* 1988; 297: 1086–1091.

34 National High Blood Pressure Education Program Working Group on Hypertension and Renal Disease. 1995 update of the working group reports on chronic renal failure and renovascular hypertension. *Arch Intern Med* 1996; 156: 1938–1947.

35 Bangstad HJ, Try K, Dahl-Jorgensen K *et al.* New semiquantitative dipstick test for microalbuminuria. *Diabetes Care* 1991; 14: 1094–1097.

36 Nelson RG, Knowler WC, Pettitt DJ *et al.* Prediction of diabetic nephropathy from untimed urine specimens. *Arch Intern Med* 1991; 151: 1761–1765.

37 Messent JWC, Elliott TG, Hill RD *et al.* Prognostic significance of microalbuminuria in insulin-dependent diabetes mellitus: a twenty three year follow-up study. *Kidney Int* 1992; 41: 836–839.

38 Mogensen CE. Prediction of clinical diabetic nephropathy in IDDM patients. Alternatives to microalbuminuria? *Diabetes* 1990; 39: 761–767.

39 Parving HH, Hommel E, Mathiesen E *et al.* Prevalence of microalbuminuria, arterial hypertension, retinopathy and neuropathy in patients with insulin dependent diabetes. *BMJ* 1988; 296: 156–160.

40 Schmitz A, Vaeth M. Microalbuminuria: a major risk factor in non-insulin-dependent diabetes: a 10 year follow-up study of 503 patients. *Diabetic Med* 1988; 5: 126–134.

41 Damsgaard EM, Froland A, Jorgensen OD *et al.* Eight to nine year mortality in known non-insulin dependent diabetics and controls. *Kidney Int* 1992; 41: 731–735.

42 Mogensen CE, Hansen KW, Osterby R *et al.* Blood pressure elevation versus abnormal albuminuria in the genesis and prediction of renal disease in diabetes. *Diabetes Care* 1992; 15: 1192–1204.

43 Krans HMJ, Porta M, Keen H. *Diabetes Care and Research in Europe: the St Vincent Declaration Action Programme.* Copenhagen: World Health Organization, 1992.

44 Hypertension in Diabetes Study (HDS). 1. Prevalence of hypertension in newly presenting type 2 diabetic patients and the association with risk factors for cardiovascular and diabetic complications. The Hypertension in Diabetes Study Group. *J Hypertens* 1993; 11: 309–317.

45 The UK Prospective Diabetes Study (UKPDS). IX. Relationships of urinary albumin and *N*-acetylglucosaminidase to glycaemia and hypertension at diagnosis of type 2 diabetes mellitus and after 3 months' of diet therapy. UK Prospective Diabetes Study Group. *Diabetologia* 1993; 36: 835–842.

46 Hansson L, Zanchetti A, Carruthers SG *et al.* for the HOT Study Group. Effects of intensive blood pressure lowering and low-dose aspirin in patients with hypertension: principal results of the Hypertension Optimal Treatment (HOT) randomised trial. *Lancet* 1998; 351: 1755–1762.

47 UK Prospective Diabetes Study Group. Efficacy of atenolol and captopril in reducing risk of macrovascular and microvascular complications in type 2 diabetes: UKPDS 39. *BMJ* 1998; 317: 713–720.

48 1999 World Health Organisation-International Society of Hypertension guidelines for the management of hypertension. *J Hypertens* 1999; 17: 151–183.

49 Pollare T, Lithell H, Berne C. A comparison of the effects of hydrochlorothiazide and captopril on glucose and lipid metabolism in patients with hypertension. *N Engl J Med* 1989; 321: 868–873.

50 Pollare T, Lithell H, Selinus I *et al.* Sensitivity to insulin during treatment with atenolol and metoprolol: a randomized double blind study of effects on carbohydrate and lipoprotein metabolism in hypertensive patients. *BMJ* 1989; 298: 1152–1157.

51 American Diabetes Association: clinical and practice recommendations. *Diabetes Care* 1997; 20 (Suppl. 1): S1–S70.

52 Curb JD, Pressel SL, Cutler JA *et al.* for the Systolic Hypertension in the Elderly Program Cooperative Research Group. Effect of diuretic-based antihypertensive treatment on cardiovascular disease risk in older diabetic patients with isolated systolic hypertension. *JAMA* 1996; 276: 1886–1892.

53 Gall MA, Rossing P, Slott P *et al.* Prevalence of micro- and macroalbuminuria, arterial hypertension, retinopathy and large vessel disease in European type 2 (non-insulin dependent) diabetic patients. *Diabetologia* 1991; 34: 655–661.

54 Schmitz A, Veath M. Microalbuminuria: a major risk factor in non-insulin-dependent diabetes. A 10-year follow-up study of 503 patients. *Diabet Med* 1987; 5: 126–134.

55 Lewis EJ, Hunsicker LG, Bain RP, Rhode RD. The effect of angiotensin-converting enzyme-inhibition on diabetic nephropathy. *N Engl J Med* 1993; 329: 1456–1462.

56 Bakris GL. Effects of diltiazem or lisinopril on massive proteinuria associated with diabetes mellitus. *Ann Intern Med* 1990; 112: 701–702.

57 Bakris GL. Hypertension in diabetic patients: an overview of interventional studies to preserve renal function. *Am J Hypertens* 1993; 6: 140S–147S.

58 Makis DD, Ma JZ, Louis TA, Kasiske BL. Long-term effects of antihypertensive agents on proteinuria and renal function. *Arch Intern Med* 1995; 155: 1073–1080.

59 Kloke HJ, Wetzels JF, van Hamersvelt HW *et al.* Effects of nitrendipine and cilazapril on renal hemodynamics and albuminuria in hypertensive patients with chronic renal failure. *J Cardiovasc Pharmacol* 1990; 16: 924–930.

60 Kamper AL, Strandgaard S, Leyssac PP. Effect of enalapril on the progression of chronic renal failure. A randomized controlled trial. *Am J Hypertens* 1992; 5: 423–430.

61 Mann JF, Reisch C, Ritz E. Use of angiotensin-converting enzyme inhibitors for the preservation of kidney function. *Nephron* 1990; 55 (Suppl. 1): 38–44.

62 Ravid M, Lang R, Radimani R, Lishner M. Long term renoprotective effect of angiotensin-converting enzyme inhibition in noninsulin dependent diabetes mellitus: a 7 year follow-up study. *Arch Intern Med* 1996; 156: 286–289.

63 Sano T, Kawamura T, Matsumae H *et al.* Effects of long-term enalapril treatment on persistent microalbuminuria in well-controlled hypertensive and normotensive NIDDM patients. *Diabetes Care* 1994; 17: 420–424.

64 Ferrari P, Rosman J, Weidmann P. Antihypertensive agents, serum lipoproteins and glucose metabolism. *Am J Cardiol* 1991; 67: 26–35.

65 The Treatment of Mild Hypertension Research Group. The treatment of mild hypertension study. A randomized, placebo-controlled trial of nutritional-hygienic regimen with various drug monotherapies. *Arch Intern Med* 1991; 151: 1413–1423.

66 Lehtonen A, and the Finnish Multicenter Study Group. Lowered levels of serum insulin, glucose and cholesterol in hypertensive patients during treatment with doxazosin. *Curr Ther Res* 1990; 47: 278–282.

67 Stamler R, Stamler J, Gosch FC *et al.* Initial antihypertensive drug therapy: a comparison of α-blocker (prazosin) and diuretic (hydrochlorothiazide). *Am J Med* 1989; 86 (Suppl. 1B): 24–27.

68 Pollare T, Lithell H, Selinus I *et al.* Application of prozosin in association with an increase in insulin sensitivity in obese patients with hypertension. *Diabetologia* 1988; 31: 415–420.

69 Scandinavian Simvastatin Survival Study Group. Randomized trial of cholesterol lowering in 4444 patients with coronary heart disease: the Scandinavian Simvastatin Survival Study (4S). *Lancet* 1994; 344: 1383–1389.

70 Reaven GM. Banting Lecture: role of insulin resistance in human disease. *Diabetes* 1988; 37: 1595–1607.

71 Reaven GM. Role of insulin resistance in human disease (Syndrome X): an expanded definition. *Ann Rev Med* 1993; 44: 121–131.

72 Frayn KN. Insulin resistance and lipid metabolism. *Curr Opin Lipidol* 1993; 4: 197–204.

73 Taskinen M-R. Strategies for the diagnosis of the metabolic syndrome. *Curr Opin Lipidol* 1993; 4: 434–443.

74 Leyva F, Godsland IF, Ghatei M *et al.* Hyperleptinemia as a component of a metabolic syndrome of cardiovascular risk. *Arterioscl Thromb Vasc Biol* 1998; 18: 928–933.

75 Després J-P, Marette A. Relation of components of insulin resistance syndrome to coronary disease risk. *Curr Opin Lipidol* 1994; 5: 274–289.

76 Godsland IF, Stevenson JC. Insulin resistance: syndrome or tendency? *Lancet* 1995; 346: 100–103.

8: Dyslipidaemia

The link between elevated serum cholesterol and atherosclerosis is well established [1–3]. Hypercholesterolaemia is a major modifiable risk factor for coronary heart disease (CHD), the leading cause of death in industrialized nations. In population studies, the relationship between plasma cholesterol and CHD is continuous [4], having no threshold (Fig. 8.1). Importantly, the presence of angiographically defined CHD also correlates with serum levels of total cholesterol, as well as low-density lipoprotein (LDL)-cholesterol [5–7]. It is from evidence such as this that recommendations for cholesterol lowering therapy arose [8,9]. On the basis of current evidence, treatment of dyslipidaemia in a hypertensive patient should be considered as important as treatment of hypertension *per se*.

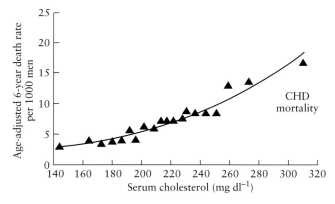

Figure 8.1 The linear relationship between plasma cholesterol and cardiovascular risk. Reproduced from [2] with permission of The Lancet Ltd.

GENETIC DYSLIPIDAEMIA

Genetic hyperlipidaemias are by no means rare, and should always be considered in patients with:
- Early onset CHD;
- Family history of early CHD, or hyperlipidaemia;

- Total cholesterol levels > 8 mmol l^{-1};
- Triglycerides > 5 mmol l^{-1};
- Xanthelasmata and cutaneous xanthomata (remnant, or type III, hyper-lipidaemia);
- Pancreatitis (familial hypertriglyceridaemia and recessively inherited lipoprotein lipase deficiency).

These conditions were previously classified by Fredrickson, but have now been re-classified according to the genetic–metabolic cause (Table 8.1). Patients with genetic dyslipidaemias are best referred to and managed in lipid specialist centres, where more detailed phenotype and genotype characterization [10] are available. Screening of immediate relatives of patients with such disorders is advisable. Signs, such as a hyperlipidaemic arcus, xanthelasmata and xanthomata, may be apparent on examination.

Table 8.1 Genetic–metabolic classification of hyperlipidemia.

Familial hypercholesterolaemia
Familial defective apoB
Familial combined hyperlipidaemia
Remnant (type III) hyperlipidaemia
Common hypercholesterolaemia
Familial hypertriglyceridaemia
Familial apolipoprotein C-II deficiency
Familial lipoprotein lipase deficiency
HDL hypercholesterolaemia

SECONDARY DYSLIPIDAEMIA

When dyslipidaemia occurs as a result of another clinical condition (Table 8.2), it is referred to as secondary. Such conditions are usually evident on clinical examination and routine investigations.

Table 8.2 Causes of secondary dyslipidaemia.

Pregnancy
Poorly controlled diabetes
Hypothyroidism
Nephrotic syndrome
Alcohol abuse
Chronic cholestasis
Renal disease
Anorexia nervosa and bulimia
Systemic lupus erythematosus
Metabolic disorders
Steroid therapy
Retinoids
Non-cardioselective β-blockers

POLYGENIC DYSLIPIDAEMIA

Unlike the genetic or metabolic dyslipidaemias, the dyslipidaemia which is found in association with CHD, hypertension and diabetes follows no clear relationship to genes or to discrete metabolic disturbances.

DIAGNOSIS

The diagnosis of dyslipidaemia can only be made by measuring circulating lipids. Dyslipidaemia may be suspected following the finding of raised cholesterol or triglycerides on a random blood sample taken at the initial visit in the hypertension clinic or in health screening clinics. The reasons for additional investigations (Table 8.3) are:
• To confirm the diagnosis of dyslipidaemia;
• To identify related conditions, such as cardiac disease, hypertension and diabetes mellitus;
• To exclude the possibility of genetic and secondary dyslipidaemia.

What and when to test
Hospital laboratories should all now provide the additional measurements of LDL- and high-density lipoprotein (HDL)-cholesterol and triglycerides. Because of quality assurance, all lipid measurements should be carried out in an appropriately qualified laboratory. Measurement with home unvalidated kits and devices other than the industry standard should be discouraged at present.

Table 8.3 Routine initial investigations for patients with abnormal lipids on screening.

Fasting lipids (cholesterol, triglycerides, LDL- and HDL-cholesterol)

Full blood count
ESR
Biochemistry
  Sodium, potassium
  Urea, creatinine
  Calcium, phosphate
  Fasting glucose
  [Urate]†
  Thyroid function tests (TSH ± T_4)‡
  Liver function tests§
ECG

---

†Although serum urate is likely to be elevated in patients with hypertension, diabetes, dyslipidaemia or heart failure, it is a poor predictor of individual risk of coronary heart disease or stroke. It should, however, be measured if gout or urate nephrolithiasis are suspected.
‡To exclude hypothyroidism. Thyroid stimulating hormone (TSH) alone is sufficient for screening.
§To exclude occult liver disease, including primary biliary cirrhosis.
ESR, erythrocyte sedimentation rate; T_4, thyroxine.

Random test. A random total cholesterol is appropriate for screening, but more than one sample is required for the diagnosis of dyslipidaemia.

Fasting test. If the initial tests yield abnormal results, a full lipid profile, comprising total cholesterol, LDL- and HDL-cholesterol and triglycerides, should be obtained after an overnight (12-h) fast. In contrast to triglycerides, plasma cholesterol levels are not affected by a recent meal [11–13].

After MI. Acute MI is associated with an increase in triglycerides and a decrease in total cholesterol, LDL-cholesterol and HDL-cholesterol from 24 to 48 h onwards [14,15] and the levels do not return to preinfarct levels for up to 3 months [16]. Therefore, it is advisable that if lipids have not been measured within 24 h of the MI, at least 3 months should elapse before remeasurement.

Who to test

As in the management of hypertension *per se*, one should focus on those patients in whom lipid disturbances are most likely to incur mortality and morbidity and in whom effective treatment is most likely to pay dividends (Table 8.1). Because more end-organ damage occurs if lipid disorders occur in association with atherosclerosis, the clinician should focus on the following categories of patients, in order of priority:

• Clinically overt *or occult* arteriosclerotic disorders, including coronary heart disease, cerebrovascular disease, renovascular disease or peripheral vascular disease;
• Diabetes mellitus (both types I and II);
• Those who are at high risk of developing these diseases, i.e. those with cardiovascular risk factors.

Suggested frequency of screening is shown in Table 8.4.

TREATMENT THRESHOLDS AND TARGETS

In the past, we have tended to stratify CHD risk by referring solely to blood cholesterol levels. However, population-based studies demonstrate that although CHD risk increases with increasing blood cholesterol concentrations, 80% of those who develop CHD have cholesterol levels similar to those who do not [17]. In fact, most individuals with established CHD have plasma cholesterol levels, which in the past would have been considered 'acceptable'. Clearly, the level of CHD risk not so much depends on the level of cholesterol, but on its association with other CHD risk factors (Table 8.5) [18,19].

The approach of waiting for the development of CHD before using lipid-lowering treatment is no longer justified, as the first manifestation of CHD is usually catastrophic (MI in men: sudden death in 13%, heart failure in 20%, angina in 41%). Fuelled by such statistics, numerous authorities have

Table 8.4 Suggested frequency of lipid screening.

At least once a year
Any atherosclerotic disease (clinically overt or occult)
  CHD
  Peripheral vascular disease
  Cerebrovascular disease
Diabetes mellitus
Hypertension
Family history of premature CHD
Familial dyslipidaemia

Every 3 years
Obese individuals (BMI > 30 kg m^{-2})
Postmenopausal women

Every 5 years
All individuals aged ≥ 20 years [12,13]

Never
Persons aged > 80 years

Table 8.5 The synergistic effect of risk factors in five hypothetical patients with different risk factor profiles.

Risk factors	Patient 1	Patient 2	Patient 3	Patient 4	Patient 5
Cholesterol (mmol l^{-1})	8.0	8.0	8.0	8.0	8.0
Triglyceride (mmol l^{-1})	1.5	1.5	1.5	1.5	4.0
HDL-cholesterol (mmol l^{-1})	1.5	1.5	1.5	1.5	0.8
Systolic blood pressure (mmHg)	120	120	120	200	200
Family history of CHD (< 60 years)	−	+	+	+	+
Smoking	−	−	+	+	+
Angina	−	−	−	−	+
Diabetes	−	−	−	−	+
Absolute risk of MI from 50–59 years (%)	5	7	30	52	100

Absence (−) or presence (+) of risk factor. Absolute risk was calculated using Boehringer Mannheim's 'Spirit Plus' calculator [18], which employs an algorithm based on the PROCAM study for cardiovascular disease in German men and women. Adapted with permission from [19].

provided guidelines on the assessment and management of blood cholesterol levels in individuals with and without CHD, i.e. for the primary and secondary prevention of CHD. Management guidelines are broadly consistent, and all coincide with an aggressive approach to lipid-lowering treatment in patients with atherosclerotic disease. There are, however, subtle differences, particularly with regard to the level of blood cholesterol at which therapy should be commenced and the target levels to be achieved. Moreover, some guidelines do not specify treatment for certain situations, for example, how one should manage cholesterol levels in individuals with asymptomatic atherosclerosis.

In addition, some guidelines do not incorporate recommendations on LDL- and HDL-cholesterol or triglyceride levels. Subtle differences between published guidelines should not cloud the central issues upon which they all agree. Recommended treatment thresholds are shown in Fig. 8.2 (identical to Fig. 4.2).

PHARMACOLOGICAL TREATMENT OF HYPERCHOLESTEROLAEMIA

Early primary prevention trials on cholestyramine [20], gemfibrozil [21] and clofibrate [22] demonstrated that reducing plasma cholesterol by ≈ 10% could reduce coronary events. However, reductions in plasma cholesterol and events were modest, and concern emerged following the finding in these studies of increases in non-cardiac mortality from cancer, trauma and suicide. The ensuing scepticism on lipid-lowering treatment, however, has now been quashed. Recent well-designed double-blind, placebo-controlled trials have shown that 'statins' are not only effective at reducing blood cholesterol levels, but also reduce coronary events and cardiovascular mortality in individuals with and without CHD, without increasing non-cardiac mortality. In fact, such trials have provided new definitions of dyslipidaemia. On the basis of current evidence, drug therapy of dyslipidaemia (with statins) should be considered as important as drug treatment for mild or moderate hypertension [23].

Statins
Statins are the drugs of choice for the treatment of the dyslipidaemia associated with hypertension, atherosclerosis and diabetes mellitus. They are clearly superior to all other lipid-lowering drugs at reducing plasma cholesterol levels.

Effects. As inhibitors of 3-hydroxy-3-methylglutaryl coenzyme A (HMG-CoA) reductase, statins inhibit the rate-limiting enzyme of cholesterol synthesis in the liver, reducing hepatic production of LDL and increasing the expression of hepatic LDL receptors, thus reducing circulating LDL levels. An increased uptake of plasma lipoproteins into the liver is mediated by an increase in the expression of cell membrane LDL receptors. Statins also increase clearance of very low-density lipoprotein (VLDL) and intermediate-density lipoprotein (IDL) particles [24]. Simvastatin and pravastatin produce typical reductions of around 25% in total cholesterol. In addition, statins produce modest falls in triglycerides and elevations in HDL-cholesterol.

The effects of simvastatin and pravastatin on plasma cholesterol and cardiovascular events are shown in Table 8.6 [25–27]. Importantly, reductions in cardiovascular events and mortality in these trials were achieved in

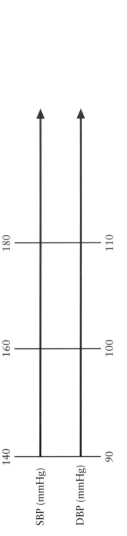

SBP (mmHg)   140   160   180

DBP (mmHg)   90   100   110

RISK STRATIFICATION

	LOW RISK	MEDIUM RISK	HIGH RISK
No risk factors, TOD or ACC	LOW RISK	MEDIUM RISK	HIGH RISK
Up to 2 risk factors	MEDIUM RISK	MEDIUM RISK	V HIGH RISK
≥ 3 risk factors ±TOD, ACC or diabetes or black race*	HIGH to V HIGH RISK	HIGH to V HIGH RISK	HIGH to V HIGH RISK

Risk of a major cardiovascular event occurring in the following 10 years: low, < 15%; medium, 15–20%; high, 20–30%; very high, ≥ 30%.

TREATMENT GOALS

ABSOLUTE RISK GROUP	BLOOD PRESSURE GOAL	LIPID GOAL	ASPIRIN
LOW RISK	Continue to monitor if: SBP > 140 ≤ 150 mmHg or DBP > 90 ≤ 95 mmHg Start drug treatment if SBP ≥ 150 mmHg or DBP ≥ 95 mmHg Aim for: BP ≤ 140/90 mmHg over 6 months	Continue to monitor total and LDL-cholesterol Aim for:	
MEDIUM RISK	Aim for: BP ≤ 140/90 mmHg over 6 months	Total cholesterol < 5.0 mmol l⁻¹ LDL-cholesterol < 3.0 mmol l⁻¹ with lifestyle advice and statins	Aspirin 75 mg o.d. for life to all treated, well controlled hypertensive patients
HIGH to V HIGH RISK	Aim for: BP ≤ 130/85 mmHg over 3 months	over 6 months	

Risk factors used for risk stratification are:
- Age: Men > 55 years, women > 65 years
- Smoking
- Total cholesterol > 6.5 mmol l^{-1} (250 mg dl^{-1})
- Family history of premature cardiovascular disease

Target Organ Damage includes:
- Left ventricular hypertrophy
- Proteinuria and/or elevation in plasma creatinine
- Ultrasound or radiological evidence of atherosclerosis
- Generalized or focal narrowing of the retinal arteries

Associated Clinical Conditions include:
- Cerebrovascular disease (ischaemic or haemorrhagic stroke or transient ischaemic attack)
- Heart disease (MI, angina, coronary revascularization, congestive heart failure)
- Renal disease (diabetic nephropathy, renal impairment)
- Vascular disease (including aortic aneurysm)
- Advanced hypertensive retinopathy (haemorrhages, exudates or papilloedema)

Figure 8.2 Diagnostic and treatment thresholds. The risk stratification table is largely based on that adopted by the 1999 WHO-ISH guidelines. It has been simplified by amalgamating the group with '3 or more risk factors or TOD or diabetes' and the group with 'associated clinical conditions' into one group. Accordingly, the risk pertaining to this group is now quoted as high-to-very high. *On the basis that in African Americans, compared to the general population, hypertension develops at an earlier age, becomes more severe, and is associated with an 80% mortality from stroke, a 50% higher mortality from heart disease, and a 320% greater rate of target organ damage, black race has been added to the group with '3 or more risk factors or TOD, or ACC or diabetes'.

Table 8.6 Trials of statins in the prevention of MI.

Study	Subjects	Age of subjects (years)	Duration (years)	Situation	Drug used	Baseline TC (mmol l⁻¹)	Reduction in TC (%)	Reduction in LDL-C (%)	Significant outcomes*
4S [25]	3617 men 827 women	35–40	4.9–6.3	Secondary prevention	Simvastatin 20–40 mg o.d.	5.5–8.0	25	35	↓ Overall mortality by 30% ↓ CHD deaths by 42% ↓ Coronary events by 34%
CARE [26]	3583 men 576 women	21–75	4.0–6.2	Secondary prevention	Pravastatin 40 mg o.d.	< 6.2	20	28	↓ Coronary events by 24% ↓ Revascularization events by 27%
LIPID [28]	7498 men 1516 women	31–75	6.1	Secondary prevention	Pravastatin 40 mg o.d.	4.0–7.0	18	25	↓ Overall mortality by 22% ↓ Revascularization events by 20% ↓ Fatal and non-fatal MI by 24%
WOSCOPS [27]	6595 men	45–64	4.9 (mean)	Primary prevention	Pravastatin 40 mg o.d.	> 6.5	20	26	↓ Cardiovascular deaths by 32% ↓ Coronary events by 31%

*$P < 0.05$ in all results shown.

TC, total cholesterol; LDL-C, low-density lipoprotein cholesterol.

Table 8.7 Extrapolation of the results of the 4S study [25], to a group of 100 patients with coronary heart disease (CHD)*.

Simvastatin 20–40 mg over median of 5.4 years	No simvastatin
Prevention of CHD death in 4	CHD in 9
Prevention of non-fatal MI in 7	Non-fatal MI in 21
Prevention of revascularization in 6	Revascularization needed in 19

*From [30] with permission of Lippincott Williams & Wilkins, Philadelphia, PA.

patients with modest levels of plasma cholesterol (5.5–8.0 mmol l⁻¹ in the 4S study [25], 6.2 mmol l⁻¹ in the CARE study [26] and 4.0–7.0 mmol l⁻¹ in the LIPID study [28]). A pooled analysis of coronary angiographic and carotid ultrasound studies with pravastatin revealed that a reduction of 52% in major coronary events paralleled a reduction in LDL-cholesterol of 28% ($p = 0.006$) [29]. Extrapolations of these studies to clinical practice (Table 8.7) pose a considerable challenge to the apparent reluctance of some physicians to use statins in patients with CHD [25,30].

The relatively early reduction in mortality seen in clinical trials of statins cannot be explained on the basis of LDL-dependent reduction in plaque volume, plaque lipid and regression of coronary atherosclerosis [31]. This suggests that the beneficial effects of statins are not solely a result of their actions on lipid metabolism but perhaps of their additional effects on vascular endothelial function, immune function, macrophage metabolism and cell proliferation. This is currently a research issue.

Cautions and adverse effects. Nausea, constipation, diarrhoea and headache are uncommon.

Raised creatine kinase (CK) levels may occur, sometimes with attending myositis and muscle pain. No cases of myositis were seen in 2081 patients treated with pravastatin [26]. Statins should be discontinued if CK levels increase to three times normal. Rhabdomyolysis is rare (1/100 000 treatment years [32]). The risk of muscle damage is higher in the case of co-existent renal impairment, hypothyroidism, or concomitant treatment with immunosuppressants (cyclosporin), fibrates or nicotinic acid.

Increased anticoagulant effects of coumarin have been observed when used concurrently with simvastatin, but not with pravastatin or fluvastatin.

Contra-indications. Breast-feeding, porphyria, active liver disease, unexplained elevations of serum transaminases. Statins are probably best avoided in children and in people who abuse alcohol. Pregnancy should be avoided during and for at least 1 month after treatment with a statin.

Choice. Although the statins do have 'class effects', it would be erroneous to assume that they are therapeutically equivalent. They certainly differ in respect of lipid-lowering efficacy [33–37] and preliminary evidence suggests that they may have varying effects on the vascular endothelium. On the basis of this and other findings, it would be unwise to assume that statins which have not been studied in morbidity and mortality trials have the same effect on these endpoints as those which have been studied. Such decisions are best taken if and when head-to-head comparisons of statins emerge from clinical outcome studies. Atorvastatin is the most potent agent, reducing plasma cholesterol by about 60% and triglycerides by 45% [38]. However, no clinical outcome trials have been carried out to explore whether reductions in plasma lipids to the levels achieved by atorvastatin translate to commensurate reductions in morbidity and mortality.

Preference. Simvastatin and pravastatin.

Dose. Starting doses of *simvastatin 20 mg o.d.* and *pravastatin 40 mg o.d.*

Follow-up. Doses can be doubled at monthly intervals until the target cholesterol level is achieved.

TREATMENT OF HYPERTRIGLYCERIDAEMIA AND LOW HDL-CHOLESTEROL

Hypertriglyceridaemia

The link between hypertriglyceridaemia and CHD is less clear-cut than for hypercholesterolaemia. There is, however, consistent evidence that hypertriglyceridaemia contributes to CHD risk, as well as to the risk of developing diabetes [39]. No studies have specifically explored whether reductions in plasma triglyceride levels translate to reductions in cardiovascular morbidity or mortality. On balance, however, the combination of plasma triglycerides > 2.3 mmol l⁻¹ and HDL-cholesterol < 0.9 mmol l⁻¹ should be treated as high risk.

In patients without CHD, fasting triglyceride levels between 2.3 and 4.6 mmol l⁻¹ should be treated initially with dietary modification. Atorvastatin is more effective than simvastatin or pravastatin at reducing triglyceride levels [40,41]. A combination of a statin and a fibrate may be required if triglyceride levels remain > 5.0 mmol l⁻¹ after non-pharmacological measures. It should be noted that high triglyceride levels carry a significant risk of pancreatitis.

Administration of ω-3 marine oils should be considered in severe hypertriglyceridaemia. It should be noted, however, that suggestions that fish oils [α-linolenic acid, eicosapentaenoic acid (EPA) and docosahexaenoic acid

(DHA)] might protect against heart disease [42,43] have not been addressed in sufficiently large studies. Resins tend to increase triglycerides and should therefore be avoided in patients with hypertriglyceridaemia.

Low HDL-cholesterol

In a *post hoc* analysis of the Helsinki Heart Study, a primary prevention study using gemfibrozil [21], the increase in HDL-cholesterol was the strongest predictor of reductions in cardiovascular events. No drug treatment is required if HDL-cholesterol rises above 0.9 mmol with weight loss, increased physical activity and dietary measures. If levels are still < 0.9 mmol l-1 and LDL-cholesterol levels remain > 2.5 mmol l-1, use of a statin or a fibrate should be considered.

High lipoprotein (a). This is an LDL-like molecule that contains apolipoprotein (a) and which shares some sequence homology with fibrinogen. Although in some populations high lipoprotein (a) levels are associated with increased CHD risk [44], no studies have addressed whether a therapeutic reduction in plasma levels translates to improvements in mortality or morbidity from CHD. Nicotinic acid is the only agent that has so far been shown to reduce lipoprotein (a) levels.

OESTROGEN REPLACEMENT THERAPY

Short-term studies have shown that oral oestrogen lowers LDL-cholesterol by 14–20% and raises HDL-cholesterol by 15–20%, although the oral forms also increase serum triglycerides by 24–38% [45]. There is considerable data from observational studies in favour of the use of oestrogen replacement therapy in the prevention of CHD in postmenopausal women. However, the HERS study, in which 2763 postmenopausal women with CHD were randomized to 0.625 mg of conjugated equine oestrogen or placebo, failed to show a reduction in CHD events by oestrogen after 4.1 years of follow up. This study has been criticized on the grounds that the dose of oestrogen used was too high. The remaining uncertainty as to whether oestrogen replacement therapy should be used in women with CHD should be resolved by ongoing studies.

LIPID EFFECTS OF ANTIHYPERTENSIVE DRUGS

In a recent meta-analysis of randomized trials, antihypertensive treatment was shown to reduce coronary events by 14%, falling short of the reversal of 20–25% predicted by prospective observational studies. There is evidence to suggest that this shortfall may be a result of the fact that diuretics and β-blockers produce an untoward risk factor profile, including the lipid

Table 8.8 Effects of antihypertensive drugs on lipids.

Drug	TC	TG	HDL-C
Diuretics*	↑3–11%	↑10–20%	→
β-blockers	↑0–5%	↑8–25%	↓5–20%
α-blockers	↓4%	↓8%	↑4%
Calcium channel blockers	→	→	→
ACE inhibitors	→	→	→
Angiotensin II receptor blockers	→	→	→

*The effects of diuretics on total cholesterol and triglycerides are dose dependent [51].
↑, increase, ↓, decrease, →, no change.
TC, total cholesterol; TG, triglycerides; HDL-C, high-density lipoprotein cholesterol.
(Adapted with permission from Opie & Frishman. *Drugs for the Heart*. 4th edn. Philadelphia: Saunders, 1995: 292.)

profile. Because one of the prime aims of treating hypertension is to improve total and cardiovascular mortality, attention to concurrent cardiovascular risk factors should be an integral part of antihypertensive management. In this respect, it is noteworthy that even a 1% reduction in total cholesterol produces detectable 1% change in all-cause mortality [47] (equivalent to a mean reduction of 0.06 mmol l⁻¹ in a population with a mean cholesterol of 6 mmol l⁻¹).

As shown in Table 8.8, treatment with α-blockers is associated with a better lipid profile than treatment with diuretics and β-blockers. Some studies have shown that the beneficial effect of prazosin [48] and doxazosin [49] over thiazides persists after 1 year of treatment. Other studies have shown that doxazosin corrects the lipid abnormalities associated with diabetes mellitus [50].

The ability of α-blockers to reduce total and LDL-cholesterol and triglycerides and to increase HDL-cholesterol makes them an appropriate choice in patients with dyslipidaemia and/or diabetes mellitus.

References

1   Kannel WB. Hypertension, blood lipids and cigarette smoking as co-risk factors for coronary heart disease. *Ann NY Acad Sci* 1978; 304: 128–139.
2   Martin MJ, Hulley SB, Bowmer WS, Kuller LH, Wentworth D. Serum cholesterol, blood pressure, and mortality: implications from a cohort of 361 662 men. *Lancet* 1986; 2: 933–939.
3   Neaton JD, Blackburn H, Jacobs D *et al.* Serum cholesterol level and mortality findings from men screened in the Multiple Risk Factor Intervention Trial. *Arch Intern Med* 1992; 152: 1490–1500.
4   Stamler J. Established major coronary risk factors. In: Marmot M, Elliot P, eds. *Coronary Heart Disease Epidemiology*. Oxford: Oxford University Press, 1992: 35–66.

5 Romm PA, Green CE, Reagan K, Rackley CE. Relation of serum lipoprotein cholesterol levels to presence and severity of angiographic coronary artery disease. *Am J Cardiol* 1991; 67: 479–483.

6 Hong MK, Romm PA, Reagan K, Green CE, Rackley CE. Effects of estrogen replacement therapy on serum lipid values and angiographically defined coronary artery disease in postmenopausal women. *Am J Cardiol* 1992; 69: 176–178.

7 Schmidt SB, Wasserman AG, Muesing RA, Schlesselman SE, Larosa JC, Ross AM. Lipoprotein and apolipoprotein levels in angiographically defined coronary atherosclerosis. *Am J Cardiol* 1985; 55: 1459–1462.

8 Consensus Conference. Lowering blood cholesterol to prevent heart disease. *JAMA* 1985; 253: 2080–2086.

9 EAS Study Group. Strategies for the prevention of coronary heart disease: a policy statement of the European Atherosclerosis Society. *Eur Heart J* 1987; 8: 77–88.

10 Humphries SE. Familial hypercholesterolaemia as an example of early diagnosis of coronary artery disease. *Br Heart J* 1986; 56: 201–205.

11 Pyörälä K, DeBacker G, Graham I, Poole-Wilson PA, Wood D on behalf of the Task Force. Prevention of coronary heart disease in clinical practice. Recommendations of the Task Force of the European Society of Cardiology, European Atherosclerosis Society and European Society of Hypertension. *Eur Heart J* 1994; 15: 1300–1331.

12 National Cholesterol Education Program. Second Report of the Expert Panel on Detection, Evaluation and Treatment of High Blood Pressure in Adults (Adult Treatment Panel II). *Circulation* 1994; 89: 1333–1445.

13 European Atherosclerosis Society. Prevention of coronary heart disease: scientific back-ground and new clinical guidelines. *Nutr Metab Cardiovasc Dis* 1992; 2: 113–156.

14 Ryder RE, Hayes TM, Mulligan IP *et al.* How soon after myocardial infarction should plasma lipids be assessed? *BMJ* 1989; 289: 1651–1653.

15 Ahnve S, Angelin B, Edhag O, Berglund L. Early determination of serum lipids and apolipoproteins in acute myocardial infarction: possibility for immediate intervention. *J Intern Med* 1989; 226: 297–301.

16 Carlsson R, Lindberg G, Westin L, Israelsson B. Serum lipids four weeks after acute myocardial infarction are a valid basis for lipid lowering intervention in patients receiving thrombolysis. *Br Heart J* 1995; 74: 18–20.

17 Kannel WB, Castelli WP, Gordon T. Cholesterol in the prediction of atherosclerotic disease. New perspectives based on the Framingham Study. *Ann Intern Med* 1979; 90: 85–91.

18 Spirit Plus Manual. The new infarct risk calculator. Mannheim: Boehringer Mannheim, 1990.

19 Dunningham M. Multiple risk factors interact. *Costs and Options* 1997; 10–12.

20 Lipid Research Clinics Program. The Lipid Research Clinics Coronary Primary Prevention Trial results. I. Reduction in incidence of coronary heart disease. *JAMA* 1984; 251: 351–364.

21 Manninen V, Elo MO, Frick MH *et al.* Lipid alterations and decline in the incidence of coronary heart disease in the Helsinki Heart Study. *JAMA* 1988; 260: 641–651.

22 Heady JA, Morris JN, Oliver MF. WHO clofibrate/cholesterol trial: clarifications. *Lancet* 1992; 340: 1405–1406.

23 Corr LA, Oliver MF. The low fat/low cholesterol diet is ineffective. *Eur Heart J* 1997; 18: 18–22.

24 Gaw A, Packard CJ, Murray EF *et al.* Effects of simvastatin on apoB metabolism and LDL subfraction distribution. *Arterioscl Thromb* 1993; 13: 170–189.

25   Scandinavian Simvastatin Survival Study Group. Randomised trial of cholesterol lowering in 4444 patients with coronary heart disease: the Scandinavian Simvastatin Survival Study (4S). *Lancet* 1994; 344: 1383–1389.

26   Sacks FM, Pfeffer MA, Moye LA *et al.* The effect of pravastatin on coronary events after myocardial infarction in patients with average cholesterol levels. *N Engl J Med* 1996; 335: 1001–1009.

27   Shepherd J, Cobbe SM, Ford I *et al.* Prevention of coronary heart disease with pravastatin in men with hypercholesterolemia. *N Engl J Med* 1995; 333: 1301–1307.

28   The Long Term Intervention with Pravastatin in Ischemic Disease (LIPID) Study Group. Prevention of cardiovascular events and death with pravastatin in patients with coronary heart disease and a broad range of initial cholesterol levels. *New Engl J Med* 1999; 339: 1349–1357.

29   Byington RP, Jukema JW, Salonen JT *et al.* Reduction in cardiovascular events during pravastatin therapy: pooled analysis of clinical events of the pravastatin atherosclerosis intervention program. *Circulation* 1995; 92: 2419–2425.

30   Kjekshus J, Pedersen TR, Tobert JA. Lipid-lowering therapy for patients with or at risk of coronary artery disease. *Curr Opin Lipidol* 1996; 11: 418–427.

31   Vaughan CJ, Murphy MB, Buckley BM. Statins do more than just lower cholesterol. *Lancet* 1996; 348: 1079–1082.

32   Rhabdomyolysis associated with lipid-lowering drugs. *Curr Prob Pharmacovigil* 1995; 21: 3.

33   Pedersen TR, Tobert JA. Benefits and risks of HMG-CoA reductase inhibitors in the prevention of coronary heart disease: a reappraisal. *Drug Safety* 1996; 1: 11–24.

34   Illingworth DR, Erkelens DW, Keller U, Thompson G, Tikkanen MJ. Defined daily doses in relation to hypolipidaemic efficacy of lovastatin, pravastatin and simvastatin. *Lancet* 1994; 343: 1554–1555.

35   Illingworth DR, Tobert JA. A review of clinical trials comparing HMG-reductase inhibitors. *Clin Ther* 1994; 16: 366–385.

36   Illingworth DR, Stein EA, Knopp RH *et al.* A randomized multicenter trial comparing the efficacy of simvastatin and fluvastatin. *J Cardiovasc Pharmacol Ther* 1996; 1: 23–30.

37   Weir MR, Berger ML, Weeks ML, Liss CL, Santanello NC. Comparison of the effect on quality of life and of the efficacy and tolerability of lovastatin versus pravastatin. The Quality of Life Multicenter Group. *Am J Cardiol* 1996; 77: 475–479.

38   Bakker-Arkema RG, Davidson MH, Goldstein RJ *et al.* Efficacy and safety of a new HMG-CoA reductase inhibitor, atorvastatin, in patients with hypertriglyceridemia. *JAMA* 1996; 275: 128–134.

39   Fontbone A, Eschwège E, Cambien F *et al.* Hypertriglyceridaemia as a risk factor of coronary heart disease mortality in subjects with impaired glucose tolerance or diabetes: results of the 11 year follow-up of the Paris prospective study. *Diabetologia* 1989; 32: 300–304.

40   Dart A, Jerums G, Nicholson G *et al.* A multicentre, double-blind, one-year study comparing safety and efficacy of atorvastatin in patients with hypercholesterolaemia. *Am J Cardiol* 1997; 80: 39–44.

41   Bertolini S, Bon GB, Campbell LM *et al.* Efficacy and safety of atorvastatin compared to pravastatin in patients with hypercholesterolaemia. *Atherosclerosis* 1997; 130: 191–197.

42   Burr ML, Sweetnam PMH, Fehily AM. Diet and reinfarction (letter). *Eur Heart J* 1994; 15: 1152–1154.

43   Bairati I, Roy L, Meyer F. Double-blind randomized, controlled trial of fish-oil

supplements in prevention of recurrence of stenosis after coronary angioplasty. *Circulation* 1992; 85: 950–956.

44 Chappel DA. Hyperlipidaemia in cardiovascular disease. *Curr Opin Lipidol* 1996; 7: U193–U201.

45 Walsh BW, Schiff I, Rosner B, Greenberg L, Ravnikar V, Sacks FM. Effects of postmenopausal estrogen replacement on the concentrations and metabolism of plasma lipoproteins. *N Engl J Med* 1991; 325: 1196–1204.

46 Hulley S, Grady D, Bush T *et al.* for the Heart and Estrogen/progestin Replacement Study (HERS) Research Group. Randomized trial of estrogen plus progestin for secondary prevention of coronary heart disease in postmenopausal women. *JAMA* 1998; 280: 605–613.

47 Law MR, Thompson SG, Wald NJ. Assessing the possible hazards of reducing serum cholesterol. *BMJ* 1994; 308: 373–379.

48 Stamler R, Stamler J, Gosch FC *et al.* Initial antihypertensive drug therapy: a comparison of α-blocker (prazosin) and diuretic (hydrochlorothiazide). *Am J Med* 1989; 86 (Suppl. 1B): 24–27.

49 The Treatment of Mild Hypertension Research Group. The treatment of mild hypertension study. A randomized, placebo-controlled trial of nutritional-hygienic regimen with various drug monotherapies. *Arch Intern Med* 1991; 151: 1413–1423.

50 Lehtonen A and the Finnish Multicenter Study Group. Lowered levels of serum insulin, glucose and cholesterol in hypertensive patients during treatment with doxazosin. *Curr Ther Res* 1990; 47: 278–282.

51 Weinberger MH. Antihypertensive therapy and lipids: evidence, mechanisms and implications. *Arch Intern Med* 1985; 145: 1102–1105.

9: Hypertension in Women: Pregnancy, Oral Contraception and the Menopause

PREGNANCY

Hypertension in pregnancy is a major cause of maternal, fetal and neonatal morbidity and mortality. Hypertensive pregnant women are at risk of developing abruptio placentae, stroke, heart failure and disseminated intravascular coagulation. The fetus of a hypertensive mother is at risk of intrauterine growth retardation, prematurity and intrauterine death.

Recommendations regarding what blood pressure levels should be considered abnormal in pregnancy are based on relatively small case-controlled studies. Unlike essential hypertension in the general population, there are few clinical outcome data on the effects of antihypertensive treatment in pregnancy and no randomized comparative studies of different pharmacological treatments have been performed. Even the largest controlled studies lack statistical power to assess the impact of different pharmacological therapies on mortality. As a result, much of the evidence relating to the diagnosis and treatment of hypertension in pregnancy has emerged from collective experience. There are, consequently, wide variations in diagnostic and treatment strategies.

CARDIOVASCULAR ADAPTATIONS

Pregnancy leads to considerable haemodynamic changes (Table 9.1). Peripheral vasodilatation, mediated by nitric oxide, oestrogen and vasodilatory prostaglandins (PGI_2), is probably the primary change. The ensuing reduction in peripheral resistance is countered by a gradual increase in heart rate (by 10–20 beats min⁻¹) and stroke volume, which increase cardiac output by as much as 40% at 28–40 weeks gestation. Changes in cardiac output and peripheral resistance cause blood pressure to decrease in early pregnancy until it reaches a nadir at 22–24 weeks gestation. Thereupon, it rises to prepregnant levels towards term. In the second trimester, blood pressure falls by about 15 mmHg of that before pregnancy. In the third trimester, it returns to the prepregnancy levels. Following delivery, blood pressure falls and then rises to reach a peak at 3–4 days postpartum. The cardiovascular adaptations

126

Table 9.1 Haemodynamic changes during pregnancy.

Parameter	Trimesters		
	1st	2nd	3rd
Systolic blood pressure	↔	↓	↔
Diastolic blood pressure	↓	↓↓	↓
Heart rate	↑	↑↑	↑↑↑
Blood volume	↑	↑↑	↑↑↑
Cardiac output	↑	↑↑	↑↑↑
Systemic vascular resistance	↓	↓↓↓	↓↓

↔, no change from prepregnancy levels; small increase (↑) or decrease (↓); moderate increase (↑↑) or decrease (↓↓) ; large increase (↑↑↑) or decrease (↓↓↓). Adapted from [1] with permission of Wiley-Liss, Inc., a subsidiary of John Wiley & Sons, Inc.

in pregnancy produce a sinus tachycardia, a 'bounding' pulse, an ejection systolic flow murmur and a third heart sound.

Classification of hypertension in pregnancy

Despite recent advances, definitions and classifications of hypertension in pregnancy are largely descriptive and uninformative. If hypertension is diagnosed for the first time in pregnancy, the most important aspect of management is to control blood pressure and to look out for pre-eclampsia. Whether or not the blood pressure elevations preceded pregnancy is somewhat superfluous. Once blood pressure has been found to be elevated, the main issue is to exclude pre-eclampsia. Accordingly, hypertension in pregnancy may be classified as follows:

- Pregnancy-specific hypertension:
  Pre-eclampsia
  Pregnancy-induced hypertension
- Co-incidental (pre-existing or newly found) hypertension:
  Secondary hypertension
  Essential hypertension

The risks of hypertension in pregnancy are not so much related to the risks of elevated blood pressure but rather, to the risks of superimposed pre-eclampsia. Because pre-existing hypertension predisposes to pre-eclampsia, the approach to the finding of an elevated blood pressure in pregnancy should be dominated by careful vigilance for the development of pre-eclampsia. In some cases, the diagnosis of essential or secondary hypertension may have been made before the pregnancy. Less commonly, however, both essential and secondary hypertension may be diagnosed for the first time during pregnancy.

Blood pressure measurement

In pregnancy, posture has a considerable influence on blood pressure.

Brachial artery blood pressure is highest with the patient sitting upright, intermediate in the supine position and lowest in the left lateral position. Because of a hyperdynamic circulation, there is a greater variability in the Korotkoff phase V sound, which may occasionally reach zero. Although there is no evidence that one sound is superior to another in predicting end-organ damage, taking the phase IV sound may offer a wider margin of safety.

There is no established blood pressure threshold on which treatment should be initiated based on self-monitoring and 24-h ambulatory monitoring of blood pressure in pregnancy. Until further studies emerge, the routine use of these methods is not recommended.

Diagnostic thresholds

Considerable debate has focused on whether hypertension in pregnancy should be diagnosed on the basis of absolute levels or relative blood pressure elevations. The following thresholds are recommended:
• A single diastolic reading (phase IV) of 110 mmHg or above or two readings of 90 mmHg or above at least 4 h apart after the 20th week of pregnancy in a previously normotensive woman [2].
• A rise of 30 mmHg systolic or > 15 mmHg diastolic compared to readings taken at < 20 weeks of pregnancy [3].
• A diastolic blood pressure of > 90 mmHg before the 20th week of pregnancy suggests pre-existing or chronic hypertension.

PRE-ECLAMPSIA

After pulmonary embolism, eclampsia is the most common cause of maternal death in industrialized nations. In addition, pre-eclampsia is the most important cause of intrauterine growth retardation in singletons with no malformations. The presence of living placental tissue, be it normal or abnormal (hydatidiform mole), is *sine qua non* for its development. It has been linked to endothelial dysfunction, vasospasm, immunological and trophoblastic disturbances, and disorders of capillary permeability, but the aetiology remains unknown. It presents in the second half of pregnancy or during labour and rarely before. Pre-eclampsia can occur for the first time even up to 6 days following delivery [4]. It occurs in 2.3–5% of primigravidae [5,6], falling to 1–2% in subsequent pregnancies.

Diagnosis

The risk factors for pre-eclampsia are shown in Table 9.2. In pre-eclampsia, the appearance of signs before the appearance of symptoms is characteristic. As in the case of essential hypertension, emphasis should be placed on characterizing the hypertensive syndrome rather than trying to estimate risk by referring to the blood pressure level alone.

Table 9.2 Risk factors for pre-eclampsia.

Maternal
Age < 20 or > 35
First pregnancy
Previous severe pre-eclampsia
Family history of pre-eclampsia or
    eclampsia
Underweight and short stature
Migraines
Chronic hypertension
Chronic renal failure

Fetal
Multiple pregnancy
Hydatidiform mole
Placental hydrops

Adapted from [7].

Maternal. The features of pre-eclampsia in the mother are as follows:
• Elevated blood pressure: mild, 140/90 mmHg; severe, 170/110 mmHg.
• Visual disturbances (due to retinal ischaemia, haemorrhage and oedema).
• Nausea and right hypochondrial pain (due to stretching of the liver capsule and hepatic haemorrhages).
• Generalized (pretibial, face and hands) rather than dependent oedema. Oedema in the face and hands, however, may be present in normotensive patients (64%) in the third trimester. Conversely, up to 40% of women with eclampsia have no oedema. On this basis, some authorities recommend that oedema and weight gain should not be used to define hypertensive disorders in pregnancy.
• Vomiting and oliguria are late signs.
• Headache, and signs of increased intracranial pressure (papilloedema, hyperreflexia) are ominous signs.
• Seizures, cerebrovascular events and spontaneous bruising (disseminated intravascular coagulation) are ominous signs.

Fetal. The features of pre-eclampsia in the fetus are as follows:
• Intrauterine growth retardation.
• Asphyxia.
• Abruptio placentae (?).
In-hospital investigations should be geared towards excluding other causes of hypertension and in assessing end-organ damage. Features that might suggest pre-eclampsia are as follows:

- 4-hourly blood pressures: mild, 140/90; severe, 160/110 mmHg;
- Serial plasma urate levels: > 350 µmol l^{-1};
- Urea: > 4.5 mmol l^{-1};
- Creatinine: > 120 µmol l^{-1};
- Liver enzymes: elevated, especially AST and ALT;
- Prothrombin time: prolonged;
- Fibrinogen: < 2 g l^{-1};
- Thrombocytopenia < 100 × 10^3 mm^{-3}*;
- 24-h creatinine clearance: < 90 ml min^{-1};
- 24-h protein excretion: mild, > 0.3 g per 24 h; severe, > 2 g per 24 h†;
- 24-h excretion of adrenaline and noradrenaline metabolites increased;
- Uterine artery Doppler ultrasound: bilateral notches as at 20 or 24 weeks gestation may be the best predictor of moderate-to-severe pre-eclampsia [8];
- Cardiotocogram: signs of fetal stress.

*Thrombocytopenia may occur in up to 25% of hypertensives. The combination of Haemolysis, Elevated Liver enzyme levels and Low Platelet count constitutes the HELLP syndrome. Thrombocytopenia is a useful indicator of severity and potential for recovery.

†24-h urine collection remains the most reliable method for assessment of proteinuria. 'Dipstick' measurements are simple and rapid to perform, but the results are unreliable; positive results (1+ or greater) should be followed up with a 24-h urine collection; negative results do not rule out proteinuria.

Although serial changes in the above parameters are more informative than absolute values, the general consensus is that severe pre-eclampsia should be diagnosed if any of the following features are present [9]:

Signs of severe pre-eclampsia

- Blood pressure persistently > 160/110 mmHg
- Proteinuria > 2 g per 24 h
- Oliguria < 400 ml per 24 h
- Thrombocytopenia < 100 × 10^3 mm^{-3}
- Pulmonary oedema
- Persistent cerebral or visual disturbances
- Persistent epigastric or right upper quadrant pain

Aggressive vs. conventional management

The decision as to the timing of delivery and the choice of aggressive vs.

conservative management rests on the balance of risks for the mother and fetus [10]. Whereas aggressive management with immediate delivery is associated with extremely high neonatal mortality [11], prolongation of pregnancy exposes the mother to considerable morbidity [12]. The decision is particularly difficult between 24 and 34 weeks gestation. Despite intense efforts, the mortality from eclampsia [13,14] remains unchanged.

ANTIHYPERTENSIVE TREATMENT IN PREGNANCY

Although a statistically insignificant trend towards reducing perinatal mortality has been reported with antihypertensive treatment [15], it does not prevent the development of pre-eclampsia [16]. However, because of the loss of cerebral autoregulation and the risk of cerebral haemorrhage, blood pressure elevations should be treated regardless of the suspected underlying pathology.

Some women who are already being treated for essential hypertension may be able safely to discontinue all treatment before conception, so as to avoid early fetal exposure to the possible adverse effects of antihypertensive drugs. Those who are unable to discontinue treatment at the beginning of pregnancy may be able to do so in the second trimester, although they will be likely to require treatment in the third trimester. Against the decision of continuing antihypertensive treatment is the low maternal risk of running elevated blood pressures for 9 months. Such decisions are best taken in specialized centres. Thresholds above which antihypertensive treatment is commenced vary, although none have been rigorously assessed in relation to subsequent morbidity and mortality. There is, however, general agreement on the following:

> Pharmacological treatment should be instituted in pregnant women with systolic blood pressure greater than 169 mmHg or a diastolic pressure greater than 109 mmHg, or both [17].

Mild-to-moderate hypertension

There are wide variations in treatment thresholds and no firm recommendations can be made at present. Some recommend treatment when diastolic blood pressure is 100 mmHg or above [3], whilst others consider that treatment of blood pressure below 160/110 mmHg *without* proteinuria confers little advantage to mother or fetus [18]. Each case must clearly be judged on the basis of perceived risks and benefits of antihypertensive treatment. The drugs available for treatment of mild-to-moderate hypertension in pregnancy are shown in Table 9.3.

Table 9.3 Drugs and doses used in the treatment of mild-to-moderate hypertension in pregnancy*.

Drug†	Initial dose	Maximum dose
Methyldopa	250 mg b.d.	1 g t.d.s.
Hydralazine	25 mg t.d.s.	75 mg q.d.s.
Nifedipine SR‡	10 mg b.d.	40 mg b.d.
Labetalol	100 mg b.d.	500 mg t.d.s.

*All the above drugs are considered safe during breast feeding.
†Labetalol, hydralazine and nifedipine may give rise to side-effects which may mimic fulminating pre-eclampsia (headache, tremor, nausea and vomiting).
‡Slow release oral preparation. The sublingual form of nifedipine is not adequately absorbed [19,20].

Methyldopa
Effects. Methyldopa reduces blood pressure by a central mechanism, probably involving depletion of noradrenaline and dopamine levels in the anterior hypothalamic-preoptic region and in the medulla oblongata. It has a slow onset of action (maximum blood pressure fall in 6–9 h) and therefore, is not useful in hypertensive emergencies. In chronic hypertension, it is effective [16] and its long-term safety has been assessed [21]. Although it crosses the placenta, effects on fetal heart rate and reductions in fetal blood pressure are not clinically significant. Because of its interference with catecholamine assays, it should be avoided in patients with suspected phaeochromocytoma.

Cautions and adverse effects. Daily doses of 1 g seldom produce adverse effects. Side-effects, usually when daily doses exceed 1.5 g, include nasal congestion and xerostomia, but these tend to resolve with duration of treatment. Sedation, malaise, depression and orthostatic hypotension may be more long-lasting. Hypersensitivity reactions, such as hepatitis and drug fever have been reported. Coombes-positivity is common but this is not an indication for discontinuation of treatment unless it is accompanied by haemolytic anaemia.

Doses. Methyldopa 250 mg b.d. initially, increasing to a maximum of 1 g t.d.s. according to blood pressure response.

Labetalol. There is concern that β-blockers may affect fetal growth when started before the 28th week of pregnancy [22,23]. This concern extends to labetalol, which combines α- and β-blocking effects when used at high doses. The latter should therefore be reserved for short-term use in the third trimester, either in combination with other agents or if patients are intolerant of methyldopa, with hydralazine and nifedipine. A history of asthma is a contra-indication to its use.

β-Blockers. Although safe in the short term, β-blockers are contra-indicated in the long-term treatment of hypertension in pregnancy, given their associations with small fetuses [22] and placentas [23]. Pregnant women with pre-existing hypertension should be changed over to methyldopa when pregnancy is diagnosed.

Diuretics. Although diuretics reduce the incidence of hypertension and oedema, they do not prevent pre-eclampsia or reduce perinatal mortality [24]. They interfere with physiological adaptations in volume expansion [18] and thus may compromise uteroplacental perfusion [3]. They should be avoided in pre-eclampsia and intrauterine growth retardation. Their use should be limited to the treatment of pulmonary oedema and pathological fluid retention — rare complications of pre-eclampsia.

Calcium antagonists. Experience with these agents is limited and some authors have expressed caution in their use in pregnancy [25]. Although a popular route of administration, the 'sublingual' route does not ensure absorption [19,20]. The slow-release oral preparation can be considered an alternative in patients who are intolerant of methyldopa and hydralazine.

ACE inhibitors. These have been associated with oligohydramnios and neonatal death from renal failure [26]. All female patients of reproductive age must be warned of this risk. Patients on maintenance therapy with ACE inhibitors for pre-existing hypertension should be switched to methyldopa when pregnancy is diagnosed.

Acute severe hypertension

An agreed management plan, involving obstetricians, intensive care specialists, paediatricians and physicians, should be drawn locally [27,28]. The aim in management is to prevent cerebral haemorrhage, cardiac failure, MI and placental abruption [29,30].

Most authorities commence urgent treatment if the blood pressure exceeds 170/110 mmHg [31]. The goal should be to achieve blood pressure control within 3 h. It is imperative to optimize cardiac preload using volume expansion, preferably with colloid and ideally with central venous and pulmonary artery pressure monitoring in the critically ill [32]. Hydralazine, administered intravenously as an infusion or as boluses, has traditionally been used [33]. Labetalol is also effective [34], although there are no data on perinatal effects. Oral rather than sublingual nifedipine (5–10 mg repeated 4–6 hourly) has been used effectively, but should be used with caution if magnesium sulphate is being administered for seizure prophylaxis, as the combination may cause profound hypotension [35]. Diazoxide should now be avoided, given the risk of profound hypotension and cerebral ischaemia [36].

ORAL CONTRACEPTION

Slight increases in systolic and diastolic blood pressure are witnessed in most women taking oral anticontraceptives. The magnitude of the blood pressure elevation appears to depend on the dose of oestrogen, being lesser at the 30 μg doses of oestrogen. A study in the 1960s revealed that compared to other women, women who took the oral contraceptive pill were up to 3 times more likely to be hypertensive, particularly if they were obese or older [37]. A recent study did not find an increased risk of stroke in women taking oestrogen at a dose of < 50 μg [38].

It is prudent to check blood pressure every 3 months after commencing oral contraceptives. If hypertension does develop, the oestrogen-based oral contraceptive must be discontinued and use of an alternative contraceptive, including the progestogen-only pill, be considered. If within 6 months of treatment blood pressure does not settle to the patient's normal blood pressure, the possibility of hypertension secondary to other causes should be contemplated.

THE MENOPAUSE

Cardiovascular disease is the most common cause of morbidity and mortality in postmenopausal women. Half will develop CHD in their lifetime, 30% will die from the disease and 20% will develop a stroke [39–41]. In contrast, only 0.3% and 3% will die of endometrial and breast cancer, respectively [41].

The menopause usually starts at around 50 years of age (range 41–59 years), although ovarian production of oestrogen and progestogen begins some years before the menses stop. Most of the important causes of morbidity in postmenopausal women, such as cardiovascular disease, osteoporosis and various cancers have been linked to the state of oestrogen deficiency that accompanies the menopause. Importantly, the age-independent increase in CHD risk which is associated with the menopause [42–46] is paralleled by metabolic disturbances similar to those found in men, and most of these have now been linked to oestrogen deficiency [47] (Table 9.4). Several disease and management-related aspects are different between the sexes (Table 9.5).

Management of hypertension in the menopause

In the large clinical trials of antihypertensive treatment, no consistent gender differences in the responses to antihypertensive treatment have emerged [62] (Table 9.6). On the basis of such studies and other clinical trials, there is no reason to suppose that antihypertensive treatment should be specifically tailored to women during the menopause.

Table 9.4 Causes of morbidity and mortality in postmenopausal women that are linked to oestrogen deficiency.

Coronary heart disease
Osteoporosis*
  Hip fracture
  Vertebral fracture

Vasomotor symptoms ('hot flushes')
Sleep disturbances and somatic symptoms
Urogenital problems
  Vulvovaginal atrophy
  Dyspareunia
  Dysuria
  Incontinence
  Urinary tract infections
  Vaginal dryness

*A 50-year-old white woman has a 16% probability of eventually suffering a hip fracture and a 32% risk of vertebral fracture [40].

Table 9.5 Features of cardiovascular disease in women compared to men.

Disease-related aspects
Atypical symptoms of MI more common, particularly in older women
Women with MI present later to hospital
Higher in-hospital mortality from MI [48,49]
More acute complications of MI [50–52], even after thrombolytic therapy [53,54]
More complications [55,56] and mortality [57] from CABG
Lower rates of CABG patency and more likely to require a second CABG [58]
More women eventually develop hypertension [59]

Management-related aspects
Less likely to receive thrombolytic treatment, β-blockers and aspirin [60]
More likely to be older, have hypertension, hypercholesterolaemia and NIDDM when referred
  to PTCA [61]
Less likely to be referred for exercise rehabilitation after MI

MI, myocardial infarction; CABG, coronary artery bypass grafting; PTCA, percutaneous transluminal coronary angioplasty.

Oestrogen replacement therapy. Oestrogen replacement therapy has a proven benefit in the relief of climacteric symptoms and in the prevention of osteoporosis. Increasing attention is being focused on the use of oestrogen replacement therapy in the prevention of CHD [64,65]. In *observational* studies of postmenopausal women, oestrogen replacement therapy is associated with a reduced incidence of CHD [66]. In the Lipid Research Clinics Program Follow-up Study, women who were selected on the basis of elevated lipid levels appeared to benefit most from oestrogen replacement [67], suggesting that oestrogen use may be more protective in women with CHD risk

Table 9.6 Mortality by sex in hypertension trials.

	No. of subjects	% women	% change in end-point	
			Men	Women
HDFP, 1979	10 940	46	Black: ↓ 18.5 White: ↓ 14.7	Black: ↓ 27.8 White: ↑ 2.5
Australian, 1980	3 427	37	↓ 26 †	↓ 36 †
MRC, 1985	17 354	48	↓ 15	↑ 26
EWPHE, 1985	840	70	↓ 47 ‡	↓ 18 ‡
SHEP, 1991	4 736	56	↓ 33 §	↓ 36 §
MRC, Elderly, 1992	4 396	58	↓ 21 ‡	↑ 11 ‡

HDFP, Hypertension Detection and Follow-up Program; MRC, Medical Research Council trial; EWPHE, European Working Party on High Blood Pressure in the Elderly Trial; SHEP, Systolic Hypertension in the Elderly Program. Reproduced from [63] with permission of the American Medical Association © 1995. ↓, Reduction; ↑, increase; †, total end-points, not mortality; ‡, cardiovascular mortality only; §, stroke events only.

factors than in those without. This is consistent with the finding from another observational study showing that women with CHD who were not using hormone replacement therapy (HRT) had a 37% lower survival than users [68]. In another study of women who underwent coronary artery bypass surgery, the 10-year survival of users of HRT was about 16% lower in users of hormone replacement therapy (HRT) compared to non-users [69]. Overall, observations indicate 37–44% reduction in risk of CHD among ever-users of oestrogen [41,66]. The HERS study [70] is the only randomized, controlled study of oestrogen replacement in women with CHD so far performed. In this study, 2763 postmenopausal women with CHD were randomized to 0.625 mg of conjugated equine oestrogen or to placebo. It showed that although oestrogen replacement led to a 11% reduction in LDL-cholesterol and a 10% elevation in HDL-cholesterol, it did not lead to a reduction in CHD events after 4.1 years of follow up. This study should not be adopted as definitive. It has been criticized on the grounds that the dose of oestrogen used was too high and that this may have been responsible for the trend towards an increase in CHD events after 1 year of treatment. Until further studies are performed, oestrogen replacement therapy should be used with caution in the secondary prevention of CHD. Nevertheless, it may be appropriate to continue therapy in women who are already receiving it, given the favourable pattern in CHD events after several years of therapy. Oestrogens, either alone or combined with progestogens, do not increase the incidence of stroke [41,71]. It is noteworthy that although transdermal preparations are effective in relieving climacteric symptoms and in preventing osteoporosis, their effects on lipids are mild, and their cardiovascular benefits remain unknown.

Cardiovascular effects of HRT. A lowering of total plasma cholesterol and triglycerides, an increase in HDL-cholesterol, and a reduction in atherogenic, oxidized LDL-cholesterol may contribute to the cardiovascular benefits of HRT. On the other hand, orally and transdermally administered oestrogens, either alone or combined with progestogens, appear to have little effect on blood pressure [72–74]. In approximately 5% of women, conjugated equine oestrogens lead to an idiosyncratic blood pressure elevation [75]. Blood pressure tends to decrease in hypertensive women treated with 17-β oestradiol [76]. On balance, HRT is safe in hypertensive women, although some women experience an elevation in blood pressure with oestrogen therapy. A 6-monthly check on blood pressure is recommended after commencing oestrogen replacement therapy.

Cautions and adverse effects. Prolonged use of unopposed oestrogens increases the risk of endometrial hyperplasia and endometrial cancer (sixfold increase in endometrial cancer among women who use oestrogen for 5–10 years) and for this reason, non-hysterectomized women should receive progestogens as well as oestrogens.

There is a modest but significant increase in the risk of breast cancer with oestrogen therapy (RR = 1.2–1.4) [77,78], although this apparent increase may be due to earlier diagnosis in the studies (i.e. surveillance bias).

Doses. The minimum effective daily dose of oestrogen is 0.625 mg conjugated oestrogen. For non-hysterectomized women, progestogen therapy is required to prevent endometrial hyperplasia and cancer. The most common progestogen regime is 2.5 mg medroxyprogesterone acetate (MPA) daily, or a cyclic regimen of 5–10 mg MPA daily for 10–14 days of each month.

Based on current evidence, oestrogen replacement therapy cannot be recommended for all postmenopausal women. The current evidence from observational studies is in favour of the use of HRT in women with established CHD who have not had breast cancer or a family history of breast cancer. However, we await the results of randomized clinical outcome studies of HRT before making evidence-based recommendations for the use of HRT in women with CHD.

References

1 Elkayam U, Gleicher N. Hemodynamics and cardiac function during normal pregnancy and the puerperium. In: Elkayam U, Gleicher N, eds. *Cardiac Problems in Pregnancy: Diagnosis and Management of Maternal and Fetal Disease*, 2nd edn. New York: Alan R. Liss, 1990: 5.

2   Davey DA, MacGillivray I. The classification and definition of the hypertensive disorders of pregnancy. *Am J Obstet Gynecol* 1988; 158: 892–898.

3   National High Blood Pressure Education Program Working Group report on high blood pressure in pregnancy. *Am J Obstet Gynecol* 1990; 163: 1691–1712.

4   Chapman KK. A case of post partum eclampsia of late onset confirmed by autopsy. *Am J Obstet Gynecol* 1973; 117: 858–861.

5   Nelson TR. A clinical study of pre-eclampsia. Part I. *J Obstet Gynaecol Br Emp* 1955; 62: 44–57.

6   Saftlas AF, Olson DR, Franks AL, Atrash HK, Pokras R. Epidemiology of preeclampsia and eclampsia in the United States 1979–86. *Am J Obstet Gynecol* 1990; 163: 460–465.

7   Redman CWG. Hypertension in pregnancy. In: Swales J, ed. *Textbook of Hypertension*. Oxford: Blackwell Scientific Publications, 1994: 767–784.

8   Aquilina J, Harrington K. Pregnancy hypertension and uterine artery Doppler ultrasound. *Curr Opin Obstet Gynecol* 1996; 8: 435–440.

9   American College of Obstetricians and Gynecologists. *Management of Severe Pre-Eclampsia*. Washington, DC: American College of Obstetricians and Gynecologists, 1986.

10 Sibai BM, Frangieh AY. Management of severe preeclampsia. *Curr Opin Obstet Gynecol* 1996; 8: 110–113.

11 Sibai BM, Mercer BM, Schiff E, Friedman SA. Aggressive versus expectant management of severe preeclampsia at 28–32 weeks' gestation: a randomized controlled trial. *Am J Obstet Gynecol* 1994; 171: 818–822.

12 Schiff E, Friedman SA, Sibai BM. Conservative management of severe pre-eclampsia remote from term. *Obstet Gynecol* 1994; 84: 626–630.

13 Sibai BM, Taslimi M, Abdella TN, Brooks TF, Spinnato JA, Anderson GD. Maternal and perinatal outcome of conservative management of severe pre-eclampsia in midtrimester. *Am J Obstet Gynecol* 1985; 152: 32–37.

14 Sibai BM. Maternal-perinatal outcome in 154 consecutive pregnancies. *Am J Obstet Gynecol* 1990; 163: 1049–1055.

15 Collins R, Duley L. Beta-blockers vs methyldopa in the treatment of preeclampsia. In: Chalmers I, ed. *Oxford Database of Perinatal Trials*, Version 1 3 Disk Issue 8. 1992.

16 Redman CWG, Beilin LJ, Bonnar J. Treatment of hypertension in pregnancy with methyldopa: blood pressure control and side effects. *Br J Obstet Gynaecol* 1977; 84: 419–426.

17 Department of Health and Social Security. *Report on Confidential Enquiries Into Maternal Deaths in England and Wales 1982–84*. London: HMSO, 1989.

18 Kyle PA, Redman CWG. Comparative risk-benefit assessment of drugs used in the management of hypertension in pregnancy. *Drug Safety* 1992; 7: 223–234.

19 Spence JD, Arnold LJMO, Gilbert JJ. Vascular consequences of hypertension and effects of antihypertensive therapy. In: Robertson J, ed. *Handbook of Hypertension*. Amsterdam: Elsevier, 1992: 621–654.

20 Van Harten J, Burggraaf K, Danhof M *et al.* Negligible sublingual absorption of nifedipine. *Lancet* 1987; ii: 1363–1365.

21 Cockburn J, Moar VA, Ounsted M, Redman CWG. Final report of study on hypertension during pregnancy: effects of specific treatment on the growth and development of the children. *Lancet* 1982; i: 647–649.

22 Sibai BM, Gonzalez AR, Mabie WC, Moretti M. A comparison of labetalol plus hospitalisation versus hospitalisation alone in the management of preeclampsia remote from term. *Obstet Gynecol* 1987; 70: 323–327.

23 Butters L, Kennedy S, Rubin PC. Atenolol in essential hypertension during pregnancy. *BMJ* 1990; 301: 587–589.

24 Collins R, Yusuf S, Peto R. Overview of randomised trials of diuretics in pregnancy. *BMJ* 1985; 290: 17–23.

25 Redman CWG. Hypertension in pregnancy. In: Swales J, ed. *Textbook of Hypertension*. Oxford: Blackwell Scientific Publications, 1994: 767–784.

26 Hanssens M, Kierse MJNC, Vankelecom F, Van Assche FA. Fetal and neonatal effects of treatment with angiotensin-converting enzyme inhibitors in pregnancy. *Obstet Gynecol* 1991; 78: 128–135.

27 Hibbard BM, Anderson MM, Drife JO *et al.* Report on Confidential Enquiries into Maternal Deaths in the United Kingdom 1991–93. In: *Scottish Office Department of Health DoHaSS, Northern Ireland*. ed. Department of Health WO. London: HMSO, 1991–1993.

28 Nelson-Piercy C. *Handbook of Obstetric Medicine*. Oxford: ISIS Medical Media, 1997.

29 Glifford RW, August PA, Chesley LC *et al.* National High Blood Pressure Education Program Working Group Report on High Blood Pressure in Pregnancy. *Am J Obstet Gynecol* 1990; 163: 1689–1712.

30 Roberts JM, Redman CWG. Pre-eclampsia: more than pregnancy-induced hypertension. *Lancet* 1993; 341: 1447–1451.

31 Lubbe WF. Hypertension in pregnancy: whom and how to treat. *Clin Perinatol* 1987; 18: 845–873.

32 Cowles T, Abdelaziz S, Cotton DB. Hypertensive disorders of pregnancy. In: James D, Steer P, Weiner C, Gonil B, eds. *High Risk Pregnancy, Management Options*. London: WB Saunders Ltd, 1996: 253–275.

33 Chamberlain GV, Lewis PJ, De Swiet M, Bulpitt CJ. How obstetricians manage hypertension in pregnancy. *BMJ* 1978; 1: 626–629.

34 Mabie WC, Gonzalez AR, Sibai BM, Amon E. A comparative trial of labetalol and hydralazine in the acute management of severe hypertension in pregnancy. *Obstet Gynecol* 1987; 70: 328–333.

35 Waisman GD, Mayorga LM, Camera MI, Vigolo CA, Matinotti A. Magnesium plus nifedipine: potentiation of hypotensive effect in pre-eclampsia? *Am J Obstet Gynecol* 1988; 159: 308–309.

36 Ledingham JGG, Rajagopalan B. Cerebral complications in the treatment of accelerated hypertension. *Quart J Med* 1979; 48: 25–41.

37 Woods JW. Oral contraceptives and hypertension. *Lancet* 1967; 2: 653–654.

38 Petitti DB, Sidney S, Bernstein A, Wolf S, Quesenberry C, Ziel HK. Stroke in users of low-dose oral contraceptives. *N Engl J Med* 1996; 335: 8–15.

39 Kuhn FE, Rackley CE. Coronary artery disease in women: risk factors, evaluation, treatment and prevention. *Arch Intern Med* 1993; 153: 2626–2636.

40 Cummings SR, Black DM, Rubin SM. Lifetime risks of hip, Colles' or vertebral fracture and coronary heart disease among white postmenopausal women. *Arch Intern Med* 1989; 149: 2445–2448.

41 Grady D, Rubin SM, Petitti DB *et al.* Hormone therapy to prevent disease and prolong life in postmenopausal women. *Ann Intern Med* 1992; 117: 1016–1037.

42 Oliver MF, Boyd GS. Effect of bilateral ovariectomy on coronary heart disease and serum lipid levels. *Lancet* 1959; 2: 690–692.

43 Sznajderman M, Oliver MF. Spontaneous premature menopause, ischaemic heart disease, and serum lipids. *Lancet* 1963; I: 962–964.

44 Rich-Edwards JW, Manson JE, Hennekens CH, Buring JE. The primary prevention of coronary heart disease in women. *N Engl J Med* 1995; 332: 1758–1766.

45 Kitler ME. Coronary disease: are there gender differences? *Eur Heart J* 1994; 15: 409–417.

46 Gordon T, Kannel WB, Hjortland MC, McNamara PM. Menopause and coronary heart disease. The Framingham Study. *Ann Intern Med* 1978; 89: 157–161.

47 Stevenson JC, Crook D, Godsland IF. Influence of age and menopause on serum lipids and lipoproteins in healthy women. *Atherosclerosis* 1993; 98: 83–90.

48 Kostis JB, Wilson AC, O'Dowd K *et al.* Sex differences in the management and long-term outcome of acute myocardial infarction. A statewide study. *Circulation* 1994; 90: 1715–1730.

49 Maynard C, Litwin PE, Martin JS, Weaver WD. Gender differences in the treatment and outcome of acute myocardial infarction. Results from the myocardial infarction triage and intervention registry. *Arch Intern Med* 1992; 152: 972–976.

50 Jenkins JS, Flaker GC, Nolte B *et al.* Causes of higher in-hospital mortality in women than in men after acute myocardial infarction. *Am J Cardiol* 1994; 73: 319–322.

51 Clarke KW, Gray O, Keating NA, Hampton JR. Do women with acute myocardial infarction receive the same treatment as men? *BMJ* 1994; 309: 563–566.

52 Adams JN, Jamieson M, Rawles JM, Trent RJ, Jennings KP. Women and myocardial infarction: agism rather than sexism? *Br Heart J* 1995; 73: 87–91.

53 Weaver WD, White HD, Wilcox RG *et al.* Comparisons of characteristics and outcomes among women and men with acute myocardial infarction treated with thrombolytic therapy. *JAMA* 1996; 275: 777–782.

54 Woodfield SL, Lundergan CF, Reiner JS *et al.* Gender and acute myocardial infarction: is there a different response to thrombolysis? *J Am Coll Cardiol* 1997; 29: 35–42.

55 Bandrup-Wognsen G, Berggren H, Harford M, Hjalmarson Å, Karlsson T, Herlitz J. Female sex is associated with increased mortality and morbidity early, but not late, after coronary artery bypass grafting. *Eur Heart J* 1996; 17: 1426–1431.

56 Khan SS, Nessim S, Gray R, Czer LS, Chaux A, Matloff J. Increased mortality of women in coronary artery bypass surgery: evidence for referral bias. *Ann Intern Med* 1990; 112: 561–567.

57 Maynard C, Weaver WD. Treatment of women with acute MI: new findings from the MITI registry. *J Myocard Ischemia* 1992; 4: 27–37.

58 King BKB, Porter LA, Rowe MA. Functional, social, and emotional outcomes in women and men in the first year following coronary artery bypass surgery. *J Wom Health* 1994; 3: 347–354.

59 Anastos K, Charney P, Charon RA *et al.* Hypertension in women: what is really known. *Ann Intern Med* 1991; 115: 287–293.

60 McLaughlin TJ, Soumerai SB, Willison DJ *et al.* Adherence to national guidelines for drug treatment of suspected acute myocardial infarction. Evidence for undertreatment in women and the elderly. *Arch Intern Med* 1996; 156: 799–805.

61 Weintraub WAS, Wenger NK, Kosinski AS *et al.* Percutaneous transluminal coronary angioplasty in women compared to men. *J Am Coll Cardiol* 1994; 24: 81–90.

62 Gueyffier F, Boutitie F, Boissel JP *et al.* for the INDANA Investigators. Effect of antihypertensive drug treatment on cardiovascular outcomes in women and men: a meta-analysis of individual patient data from randomized controlled trials. *Ann Intern Med* 1997; 126: 791–797.

63 Kaplan NM. The treatment of hypertension in women. *Arch Intern Med* 1995; 155: 563–567.

64 Stevenson JC. The metabolic and cardiovascular consequences of HRT. *Br J Clin Pract* 1995; 49 (2): 87–90.

65 Stevenson JC, Crook D, Godsland IF, Collins P, Whitehead MI. Hormone replace-

ment therapy and the cardiovascular system. Nonlipid effects. *Drugs* 1994; 47 (Suppl. 2): 35–41.

66 Stampfer MJ, Colditz GA. Estrogen replacement therapy: a quantitative assessment of the epidemiologic evidence. *Prev Med* 1991; 20: 47–63.

67 Bush TL, Barrett-Connor E, Cowan LD. Cardiovascular mortality and noncontraceptive use of estrogen in women: results from the Lipid Research Clinics Program Follow-up Study. *Circulation* 1987; 75: 1102–1109.

68 Sullivan JM, Vander Zwaag R, Hughes JP *et al.* Estrogen replacement and coronary artery disease: effect on survival in postmenopausal women. *Arch Intern Med* 1990; 150: 2557–2562.

69 Sullivan JM, El-Zeky F, Vander Zwaag R, Ramanathan KB. Oestrogen replacement therapy after coronary artery bypass surgery: effect on survival. *J Am Coll Cardiol* 1994; 23: 49A.

70 Hulley S, Grady D, Bush T *et al.* for the Heart and Estrogen/progestin Replacement Study (HERS) Research Group. Randomized trial of estrogen plus progestin for secondary prevention of coronary heart disease in postmenopausal women. *JAMA* 1998; 280: 605–613.

71 Stampfer MJ, Colditz GA, Willett WC *et al.* Postmenopausal estrogen therapy and cardiovascular disease. Ten year follow-up from the Nurses' Health Study. *N Engl J Med* 1991; 325: 756–762.

72 Barret-Connor E, Bush T. Estrogen and coronary heart disease in women. *JAMA* 1991; 265: 1861–1867.

73 The writing group for the PEPI trial. Effects of estrogen or estrogen/progestin regimens on heart risk factors in potmenopausal women: the estrogen/progestin interventions (PEPI) trial. *JAMA* 1995; 273: 199–208.

74 Lip GYH, Beevers M, Churchill D, Beevers DG. Hormone replacement therapy and blood pressure in hypertensive women. *J Human Hypertens* 1994; 8: 491–494.

75 Maschak CA, Lobo RA. Estrogen replacement therapy and hypertension. *J Repro Med* 1985; 30: 805–808.

76 Luotola H. Blood pressure and haemodynamics in postmenopausal women during estradiol 17-beta substitution. *Ann Clin Res* 1983; 15: 1–121.

77 Sillero-Arenas M, Delgado-Rodriguez M, Rodrigues-Cateras R *et al.* Menopausal hormone replacement therapy and breast cancer: a meta-analysis. *Obstet Gynecol* 1992; 79: 286–294.

78 Colditz GA, Egan KM, Stampfer MJ. Hormone replacement therapy and risk of breast cancer: results from epidemiologic studies. *Obstet Gynecol* 1993; 168: 1473–1480.

10: Secondary Hypertension

Secondary hypertension is found in up to 5% of patients with hypertension, although this will vary according to whether patients are seen in primary care centres or in specialist centres. There is no single convenient screening test for secondary hypertension, although a careful clinical assessment and routine investigations often provide clues. Certain aspects of secondary hypertension are worth considering:

• In most cases, secondary hypertension is unresponsive to conventional antihypertensive drug regimes;
• Most forms of pathology underlying cases of secondary hypertension have a worse influence on all-cause morbidity and mortality than hypertension itself;
• Some forms of pathology underlying secondary hypertension can be treated by surgical or medical means;
• Secondary hypertension can occur in patients with essential hypertension.

HYPERTENSION FROM RENAL CAUSES

End-stage renal failure is a common consequence of uncontrolled hypertension [1,2]. Conversely, a wide variety of disorders affecting the kidneys can give rise to hypertension. By the time that end-stage renal failure develops, up to 90% of patients are hypertensive [3].

The renal causes of hypertension can be broadly classified as shown in Table 10.1. A clue as to whether hypertension might have a renal basis usually emerges from the finding of an elevated plasma creatinine, micro-albuminuria/proteinuria or haematuria. Investigations aimed at identifying renal causes of hypertension are shown in Table 10.2.

Renovascular hypertension
Renal artery stenosis is the commonest renovascular cause of secondary hypertension. The main causes are as follows.

Arteriosclerosis of renal arteries. This accounts for about two-thirds of cases of renal artery stenosis. It occurs most commonly in elderly men. Associated

142

Table 10.1 Renal causes of hypertension.

Renovascular causes
Renal artery stenosis / occlusion:
  Atheroma
  Fibromuscular dysplasia
  Renal arteritis (Takayasu disease*, middle aortic syndrome, systemic vasculitides, radiation
    arteritis)
  Renal artery aneurysm (usually in association with fibromuscular dysplasia)
  Renal artery thrombosis / dissection / embolus
  External compression (phaeochromocytoma, neurofibroma, aortic dissection) (very rare)
  In association with neurofibromatosis
Renal arteriovenous fistula (e.g. following renal biopsy or trauma; congenital)
Intrarenal vascular malformation

'Renal' or parenchymal causes
Glomerulonephritis in isolation
  IgA-glomerulonephritis
  Membranous glomerulonephritis
  Focal segmental glomerulonephritis

Glomerulonephritis as part of systemic disease
  Diabetes (diabetic nephropathy)
  Systemic lupus erythematosus
  Scleroderma
  Wegener's granulomatosis
  Microscopic polyarteritis
  Henoch–Schönlein purpura

Chronic pyelonephritis
Adult polycystic kidney disease
Giant renal cysts
Interstitial nephritis due to drugs
  NSAIDs

Renal hypoplasia
Renal tumours
  Renal cell carcinoma
  Wilms' tumour
  Renin-secreting tumour

Renal tuberculosis
Radiation nephritis

'Postrenal' causes
Urinary tract obstruction
Reflux nephropathy
Hydronephrosis
Renal stones

---

*Takayasu's arteritis is relatively common in Japan, China, India and Africa, and affects mainly
women.

Table 10.2 Diagnostic procedures for hypertension of suspected renal origin.

Routine investigations
Full blood count
ESR
Biochemistry
   U+Es, creatinine, uric acid
   LFTs
   Calcium, phosphate, albumin
   C-reactive protein
   Immunoglobulin electrophoresis
   Antistreptolysin titres
   Urine
   'Dipstick' analysis for albuminuria, proteinuria, microhaematuria
   24-h urine collection: creatinine and albumin clearance
   Microscopy of urine sediment (casts, red cells, white cells, Gram stain for bacteria)
Renal ultrasound (renal size, signs of obstruction?)*

Suspected renovascular cause
Isotope imaging:
   DMSA scan
   ^{99}Tc-DTPA scan with ACE inhibitor challenge
Rapid-sequence intravenous urography
Selective renal arteriography
Intravenous digital substraction angiography
Peripheral plasma renin activity
Plasma renin estimation following captopril administration   } controversial
Renal vein renin estimation

Suspected renal parenchyma disease
DMSA scan
Renal biopsy

Suspected 'postrenal' (obstructive) cause
Intravenous urography
Computed tomography
Retrograde urography
Micturating cystourethrogram

---

*Asymmetry of renal size on ultrasonography makes renovascular hypertension more likely.
Note that the right kidney can normally be up to 1.5 cm shorter than the left.
DMSA, dimercaptosuccinic acid; DTPA, diethylenetriamine pentaacetic acid; LFTs, liver
function tests; U+Es, urea and electrolytes.

factors include advanced age, smoking, atherosclerosis elsewhere (CHD, cerebrovascular disease, peripheral vascular disease) and diabetes mellitus. It usually affects the main renal artery at its ostium, the proximal third and the first bifurcation [4]. Poststenotic dilatation and collateral formation can occur as a result. Its presence does not necessarily imply that it is the cause of hypertension — it is present in up to 50% of normotensive patients with peripheral vascular disease [5,6]. Not surprisingly, therefore, a substantial number of patients remain hypertensive after correction of renal artery stenoses.

Fibromuscular dysplasia. This accounts for about one-third of cases of renal artery stenosis. It is three times more common in women. Associated factors include smoking and atheromatous renal artery stenosis. It usually affects the right main renal artery, which develops a 'string of beads' stenosis or a single discrete stenosis, depending on the histological variant.

Diagnosis

Renal artery stenosis is almost invariably asymptomatic. Examination may reveal a renal artery bruit in more than half of patients, but this is also found in patients with aortic and renal artery atheroma without renal artery stenosis. Although the clinical features of patients with renovascular hypertension are often the same as those with essential hypertension [7], the following features may suggest renal artery stenosis:

Common presentations:
- Hypertension of early onset in patients of < 30 years of age who have no family history of hypertension
- Hypertension of recent onset in patients > 55 years of age
- Hypertension and renal impairment in patients with diabetes or atherosclerosis (coronary heart disease, stroke or peripheral vascular disease (aneurysmal aorta or intermittent claudication))
- Hypertension associated with a renal bruit, particularly if asymmetrical or if it extends into diastole
- Worsening renal function ($\uparrow$ plasma creatinine by > 20 μmol l^{-1}) after initiating ACE inhibitor therapy
- Poor response to antihypertensive drug therapy

Unusual presentations:
- Malignant hypertension, with seizures and papilloedema and heart failure
- Recurrent pulmonary oedema with normal cardiac function ('flash' pulmonary oedema)
- Polyuria, polydipsia and weight loss
- Hyponatraemia and hypokalaemia
- Proteinuria and nephrotic syndrome
- Renal infarction (loin pain and haematuria)

Investigations

There is no screening test for renovascular hypertension. Most patients have a normal serum urea and creatinine. The rapid-sequence intravenous urogram and isotope renography using ^{99}Tc-DTPA is probably the most appropriate initial investigation in hypertensive patients who have been selected on clinical grounds [8]. The gold standard is selective renal arteriography, which involves a femoral artery puncture and radio-opaque contrast medium. These investigations, which are discussed in detail by Wilkinson [8] and briefly discussed in Chapter 3, are best carried out in centres specializing in renal vascular disease.

Treatment

The details of treatment of renal artery stenosis are beyond the scope of this book and the reader is referred to the review by Wilkinson [8]. Briefly, the options are as follows:

Percutaneous transluminal angioplasty. This is the treatment of choice for most cases of renal artery stenosis. Success rates vary between 40 and 90% for atheromatous disease and between 66 and 87% for fibromuscular disease. Recurrence rates are between 15 and 20% in the first year, perhaps rising to 45% at 5 years. Mortality from the procedure varies between 1 and 2%. The results of percutaneous transluminal stenting are encouraging.

Surgical correction. This is appropriate for ostial lesions, total arterial occlusions, branch stenoses, renal artery aneurysms and previous unsuccessful angioplasty. Recurrence rates are about 20% at 7 years.

Nephrectomy. This remains an option for the patient who remains hypertensive and whose affected kidney does not contribute significantly to overall renal function.

Medical treatment. β-blockers and diuretics are the most commonly used drugs in renovascular hypertension. ACE inhibitors are best avoided, as they may precipitate renal failure. They may, however, be used with close monitoring in patients in whom correction of renal artery stenosis is not possible. Other useful drugs include calcium antagonists, methyldopa and minoxidil.

HYPERTENSION AS A RESULT OF PARENCHYMAL RENAL DISEASE

Plasma creatinine levels need not be altered in patients with hypertension secondary to renal parenchymal disease. Renin hypersecretion, in the absence of renal impairment, is apt to cause elevations in blood pressure in patients with renal parenchymal disease.

The possibility of parenchymal renal disease often arises after 'prerenal' and 'postrenal' causes of hypertension have been excluded. Details of the different parenchymal renal diseases are beyond the scope of this book. The causes are listed in Table 10.1.

HYPERTENSION FROM ENDOCRINE CAUSES

The clinical assessment and routine investigations may provide clues as to whether endocrine disease (Table 10.3) is causally involved in hypertension. An outline of the special investigations of endocrine hypertension is listed in Table 10.4. The reader is referred to more specialized literature for the management of these disorders.

Table 10.3 Endocrine causes of hypertension.

Hypothyroidism
Hyperthyroidism
Cushing's syndrome*
Phaeochromocytoma*
Acromegaly*
Mineralocorticoid-induced hypertension due to:
Primary hyperaldosteronism*
Corticosterone- or deoxycorticosterone-secreting carcinoma
Idiopathic deoxycorticosterone excess
17-α hydroxylase deficiency
11-β hydroxylase deficiency
11-β hydroxysteroid dehydrogenase deficiency
Cushing's syndrome due to:
Glucocorticoid and ACTH administration
Pseudo-Cushing's syndrome associated with excessive alcohol intake
Pituitary adenoma (Cushing's disease)
Adrenocortical adenoma / carcinoma
Ectopic ACTH secretion
Ectopic GIP secretion
Ectopic CRF secretion
McCune–Albright syndrome
Carney complex
Liddle's syndrome
Gordon's syndrome
Angiotensinogen-secreting tumour
Endothelin-secreting tumour
Porphyria

*Cause of hypertension as well as hyperglycaemia.
ACTH, adrenocorticotrophic hormone; GIP, gastric inhibitory peptide; CRF, corticotrophin-releasing factor.

DRUG-INDUCED HYPERTENSION

The possibility that hypertension is caused by prescribed or unprescribed drugs must always be taken into account in the clinical assessment. A list of drugs known to cause hypertension is given in Table 10.5. The reader is referred to more specialized literature for the management of hypertension caused by these drugs.

Table 10.4 Diagnostic procedures for hypertension of suspected endocrine origin.

Routine investigations
Full blood count
ESR
Biochemistry
  Plasma
  Sodium, potassium, urea, creatinine, uric acid
  Liver function tests
  Calcium, phosphate, albumin
  C-reactive protein
  Urine
  'Dipstick' analysis for albuminuria, proteinuria, microhaematuria
  24-h urine collection: creatinine and albumin clearance
  Microscopy of urine sediment (casts, red cells, white cells, Gram stain for bacteria)
Renal ultrasound (renal size, signs of obstruction?)

Suspected thyroid disease
Plasma thyroxine and thyroid-stimulating hormone
Thyroid antibodies

Suspected phaeochromocytoma
Plasma adrenaline and noradrenaline
24-h urine collection for
  Adrenaline
  Noradrenaline
  Hydroxymethyl mandelic acid
  Normetanephrine
Clonidine suppression test†

For localizing lesions:
  Computed tomography
  Magnetic resonance imaging
  ^{133}I-metaiodobenzylguanidine scintigraphy
  Arteriography

Suspected hyperadrenalism
Plasma cortisol (after 23:00 h)
Low-dose dexamethasone suppression test‡
Intravenous dexamethasone test§
Plasma ACTH
Metyrapone test¶

For localizing lesions:
  Computed tomography
  Magnetic resonance imaging
  Adrenocortical scintigraphy

†For the clonidine suppression test, plasma is collected for noradrenaline measurements at 1,2 and 3 h following administration of clonidine 300 μg. Whereas noradrenaline will decrease in patients with essential hypertension, no such decrease is observed in patients with phaeochromocytoma.
‡Involves oral administration of dexamethasone 0.5 mg 6-hourly for 2 days.
§Plasma ACTH (adrenocorticotrophic hormone) will be high in pituitary-dependent Cushing's syndrome, and low in glucocorticoid-producing adrenocortical tumours.
¶Metyrapone inhibits 11-β hydroxylase, causing a reduction in plasma cortisol and a rise in ACTH in pituitary-dependent Cushing's syndrome. There will be no response in patients with ectopic glucocorticoid production.

Table 10.5 Drugs which are known to affect blood pressure.

Oestrogen-based oral contraceptives	BP rises in proportion to the dose of oestrogen used, being highest with the early preparations containing 100 μg of oestrogen and least with those containing 25 μg. There is little evidence that progestogen-only preparations affect blood pressure.
Non-steroidal anti-inflammatory drugs (NSAIDs)	Hypertensive effects are modest. Reduce the antihypertensive effect of most antihypertensive drugs. Note that ~15% of people aged ≥ 65 are prescribed NSAIDs.
Adrenocorticotrophic hormone (ACTH)	BP does not rise in patients with Addison's disease.
Glucocorticoids	Prolonged treatment with doses of prednisolone < 20 mg day^{-1} may have little effect on BP. Regular BP monitoring is advised for patients with chronic steroid treatment.
Mineralocorticoids	Fludrocortisone and fluroprednisolone can cause hypertension, even in patients who are receiving these drugs for postural hypotension.
Anabolic steroids	Evidence is scanty. Patients who take these agents should be warned against their considerable risks.
Liquorice and carbenoxolone	Doses of carbenoxolone > 300 mg day^{-1} are generally required to produce hypertensive effects.
Monoamine oxidase inhibitors	Inhibit the breakdown of adrenaline and noradrenaline. Tyramine-containing foods such as meat extracts, ripe cheese and grapes, broad beans and chocolate may precipitate a hypertensive crisis.
Ephedrine	Commonly found in cold remedies.
Cyclosporin	Can cause or exacerbate hypertension. Risks are higher with increasing dose and duration of treatment.
Cocaine	Causes hypertension, headache and palpitations by increasing the availability of noradrenaline. Cocaine can also cause myocardial infarction and stroke.
Clonidine withdrawal	
Tricyclic antidepressants	
Selective noradrenaline reuptake inhibitors	

HYPERTENSION RESULTING FROM COARCTATION OF THE AORTA

Coarctation of the aorta (Fig. 10.1) usually presents in infancy or childhood. Nevertheless, it may not become symptomatic until 20–30 years of age [9]. Untreated, few survive past 30 years of age. Therefore, the condition should be considered as a cause of hypertension in patients of any age. The diagnosis is suggested by:

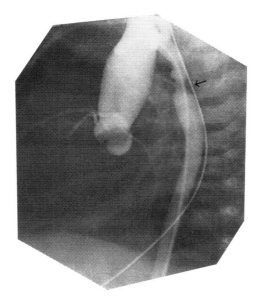

Figure 10.1 Arch aortogram in a neonate with coarctation of the aorta (arrow), distal arch hypoplasia, along with a bicuspid aortic valve and poststenotic dilatation. Figure and legend courtesy of Dr Rachel R. Phillips.

• Diminished femoral pulsations and a gap between the peak pulsation of the femoral pulse and that of the radial pulse (radiofemoral delay).
• The finding of unequal blood pressures in the upper extremities (brachial artery) compared to the lower extremities (popliteal artery). If the coarctation is proximal to the origin of the left subclavian artery, blood pressures and pulses may be different on the left and right upper limbs.
• Marked pulsations of collateral arteries over the back are sometimes present. By the time of childhood, rib-notching and cardiomegaly may be detected on the chest X-ray.
• In association with congenitally bicuspid aortic valve and patent ductus arteriosus.

Complications of aortic coarctation include cardiac failure, rupture of the ascending aorta, endocarditis and cerebral haemorrhage. Treatment is by surgical reconstruction or angioplasty. In most cases, hypertension persists despite intervention.

HYPERTENSION FROM NEUROLOGICAL CAUSES

These are extremely rare. They include:
• Intracranial tumour;
• Guillain–Barré neuropathy;
• Autonomic epilepsy.

References

1 Perry HM Jr, Miller JP, Fornoff JR *et al.* Early predictors of 15-year end-stage renal disease in hypertensive patients. *Hypertension* 1995; 25: 587–594.

2 Klag MJ, Whelton PK, Randall BL *et al.* Blood pressure and end-stage renal disease in men. *New Engl J Med* 1996; 334: 13–18.

3 Brown MA, Whitworth JA. Hypertension in human renal disease. *J Hypertens* 1992; 10: 701–712.

4 Sos TA, Pickering TG, Sniderman I *et al.* Percutaneous transluminal angioplasty in renovascular hypertension due to atheroma or fibromuscular hyperplasia. *N Engl J Med* 1983; 309: 274–277.

5 Holley KE, Hunt JC, Brown AL, Kincaid OW, Sheps SG. Renal artery stenosis. *Am J Med* 1964; 37: 14–18.

6 Dustan HP, Humphries AW, DeWolfe VG, Page IH. Normal arterial pressure in patients with renal artery stenosis. *JAMA* 1984; 187: 138–142.

7 Simon S, Franklin SS, Bleifer KH, Maxwell MH. Clinical characteristics of renovascular hypertension. *JAMA* 1972; 220: 1209–1218.

8 Wilkinson R. Renal and renovascular hypertension. In: Swales J, ed. *Textbook of Hypertension.* Oxford: Blackwell Scientific Publications, 1994: 831–857.

9 Campbell M. Natural history of coarctation of the aorta. *Br Heart J* 1970; 32: 633–638.

Part 3 Treatment of Essential Hypertension

11: Non-pharmacological Intervention

The notion that hypertension can be treated effectively by modifying lifestyle rather than with drugs is attractive for patients, doctors and public health authorities. There is sound evidence to suggest that lifestyle modifications in populations would shift the mean blood pressure level and the age-related increase in blood pressure for that population. However, no studies have shown that lifestyle modifications alone achieve clinically significant reductions in blood pressure, nor is there any evidence that such measures translate to reductions in morbidity and mortality in individual patients.

Much of the evidence that is often cited in favour of lifestyle modifications in hypertension has emerged from studies involving small numbers of subjects. Such studies have clearly shown that lifestyle modifications undoubtedly lead to changes in blood pressure and an improvement in the coronary heart disease (CHD) risk profile. However, the period of follow-up in these studies has generally been short and the lifestyle restrictions imposed on participants have been unrealistically strict. As a consequence, even persons who have agreed to take part in clinical trials, such as the TAIM study [1], have found it difficult to adhere to the study protocols.

Studies of the effects of lifestyle modifications raise inescapable difficulties for researchers, not least because it is difficult to randomize interventions. In addition, changing one lifestyle variable almost invariably changes another, e.g. lowering salt intake changes calorie intake. In the absence of randomized studies, we must rely on circumstantial evidence to arrive at the best possible advice for patients. In this respect, we should consider the evidence for the role of non-pharmacological measures in the reduction of the individual's overall CHD risk rather than rely solely on the reduction of blood pressure.

Most of the measures discussed below should be advocated in the population at large. In those with blood pressures > 180/110 mmHg, pharmacological therapy should be considered immediately. In those with lesser elevations, non-pharmacological measures should be encouraged, as they may minimize drug requirements or even obviate the need for pharmacological treatment. In addition, these measures may reduce risk of CHD independently of their effects on blood pressure lowering and the lipid profile.

SMOKING

Although there have been no randomized clinical trials on the effects of smoking on health, there is overwhelming evidence from observational studies supporting a link between smoking and an increased risk of CHD and stroke [2], as well as cancer and other diseases. Smoking triples the risk of MI, with the greatest increase in risk in women. In addition, smoking promotes renovascular and malignant hypertension and swings to high systolic pressures [3,4].

As with other cardiovascular risk factors, smoking behaves as a continuous risk variable, there being a clear dose–response relationship between the number of cigarettes smoked and CHD risk. In one study, the mortality rate from CHD in men under 65 rose from 166 per 100 000 for non-smokers to 278 for those smoking 1–14 cigarettes a day, and to 427 for those smoking 25 or more cigarettes a day [5]. Smoking potentiates cardiovascular risk in individuals with diabetes mellitus, hyperlipidaemia or hypertension. Accordingly, the death rate from CHD in a smoker with diastolic pressure greater than 90 mmHg and in the highest quantile of plasma cholesterol is about 13 times that of men in the lowest risk category.

The mechanism as to how smoking causes CHD is unclear. Increases in total cholesterol, triglycerides, LDL-cholesterol and VLDL-cholesterol, and reductions in HDL-cholesterol and apolipoprotein A1 probably contribute. Sympathetic nervous system activation, endothelial damage, altered coagulability and increased platelet aggregation have also been proposed as pathogenic factors.

Smoking should be discouraged in all individuals. Substantial reductions in cardiovascular mortality have been observed within 2 years of stopping smoking, regardless of the amount and duration of cigarette smoking or the age at which smoking is stopped [6,7]. The role of nicotine replacement and other measures [8–10] require further evaluation. Leaflets on smoking cessation may be helpful.

EXERCISE

There is little doubt that a sedentary lifestyle is associated with an increased risk of CHD, hypertension, obesity [11] and diabetes mellitus. The association between a sedentary lifestyle and hypertension [12,13] is graded [14]. As in studies of exercise in patients with CHD, randomized controlled trials of exercise in primary prevention of hypertension are limited, because they have been small, or have included other risk-modifying factors. Likewise, no studies have adequately tested whether increased physical activity leads to a reduction in the risk of developing NIDDM. It is noteworthy, however, that individuals differ in their response to the blood pressure lowering effects of exercise [15].

On balance, regular exercise moderately enhances the effects of weight reduction, produces modest reductions in blood pressure and probably improves the lipid profile.

DIETARY MEASURES

The overall aim of modifying diet in hypertensive patients is to reduce the overall risk of developing cardiovascular and non-cardiovascular disease.

Weight reduction

It is clear that morbid obesity (more than twice the desirable weight) carries increased mortality in adults [16,17]. Less severe obesity, with a body mass index in the range of 26.4–28.5 kg m^{-2} has also been associated with increased mortality in prospective cohort studies [18,19]. The health risks associated with obesity are shown in Table 11.1.

The aim of reducing weight is to reduce the amount of body fat, preferably abdominal fat. In the less overweight, weight-reducing regimens have only shown short-term efficacy and have failed to achieve long-term weight loss [17,20,21]. Long-term results of low-calorie diets have been disappointing, with most individuals returning to their prediet weight within 5 years

Table 11.1 Health risks associated with obesity.

Related to cardiovascular disease
Coronary heart disease [18,19,25,26]
Hypertension* [16,25]
Type II diabetes mellitus* [16,25,27]
Hypercholesterolaemia [16,28,29]
Stroke [30]

Other conditions
Sleep apnoea syndrome
Cancer of [25,31]:
    Colon
    Rectum
    Prostate
    Cervix
    Gall bladder
    Biliary tract
    Breast
    Endometrium
Cholelithiasis
Obstructive sleep apnoea
Venous thromboembolism
Osteoarthritis

*The prevalence of diabetes and hypertension is threefold higher in overweight adults than in adults of normal weight [32].

[22,23]. Even when combined with exercise, the degree of weight loss that can be achieved with diets is limited [22,24]. There is little point in making patients' lives miserable by submitting them to unrealistically strict measures.

Calorie notes

Average adult man uses 2500 kcal day^{-1} and an average adult woman
 2100 kcal day^{-1}
All obese people lose weight on an intake of < 1000 kcal day^{-1}
Short-term weight change is likely to reflect changes in glycogen and water
Losses greater than 1 kg per week involve loss of lean tissue rather than fat
A good cook is as important as a good dietician
Exercise is beneficial but will not, by itself, cause significant weight loss
Do not weigh more frequently than every 2–4 weeks

Lipid lowering

There is a popular belief that a low-saturated-fat, low-cholesterol diet protects against CHD. Yet, such diets have not been shown to reduce the risk of MI or all-cause mortality in primary prevention and they are conspicuously ineffective at lowering mortality in secondary prevention, as discussed by Corr and Oliver [33]. In very overweight patients (BMI = 30 kg m^{-2}), a weight reduction of 10 kg could be expected to reduce LDL-cholesterol levels by 7% and to raise HDL-cholesterol by 13% [34]. The reductions in total cholesterol that can be achieved with the American Heart Association step 1 diet are around 2–4% [35–37]. In a recent systematic overview of 19 randomized controlled trials, dietary intervention over at least 6 months was associated with a 5.3% reduction in total cholesterol [38]. Whilst, if extrapolated, such reductions would be expected to lead to significant reductions in CHD, no studies have explored this issue. In this regard, the following must be emphasized:

• It is no longer adequate to advise diet *alone* for patients with CHD [35,39].
• The effects of a low-saturated-fat, low-cholesterol diet should accompany lipid-lowering therapy, as it has additive cholesterol-lowering effects [40].
• Dietary intervention should certainly not delay treatment with statins in patients with cardiovascular or cerebrovascular disease.

Suggestions for a 'healthy diet' are shown in Table 11.2.

Reducing salt intake

Whether excessive intake of dietary salt is important in the pathogenesis of hypertension has been a long debated issue [41–46]. In contrast to experimental animal studies [47], studies within populations have failed to demonstrate a consistent relationship between blood pressure and sodium

Table 11.2 Suggestions for a healthy diet.

Food type	Eat regularly	Eat in moderation occasionally	Eat in moderation special treats	Avoid eating
Cereal food	Wholemeal flour, oatmeal Wholemeal bread, whole grain cereals, porridge oats, crispbreads, brown rice, wholemeal pasta, cornmeal, untoasted sugar-free muesli Rice cakes	White bread White flour White rice and pasta Water biscuits Wholemeal or oat scone Teacake Pancake	Sugar-coated cereals Plain semi-sweet biscuits Ordinary muesli	Sweet biscuits, cream-filled biscuits, cheese biscuits, croissants
Fruit and vegetables	All fresh, frozen, dried and unsweetened tinned fruit All fresh, frozen, dried and tinned vegetables (especially peas, any canned beans and lentils) Baked potatoes (eat skin) Tofu	Olives Oven chips labelled 'cooked in sunflower oil and 40% less fat' (grill if possible) Avocado	Fruit in syrup Crystallized fruit Chips and roast potatoes cooked in suitable oil	Deep-fat-fried chips, roast potatoes Crisps and savoury snacks
Nuts	Chestnuts Walnuts Pinenuts	Pistachio nuts. Pecans Almonds Sesame or sunflower seeds	Peanuts and most other nuts, e.g. hazelnuts, brazil nuts, cashew	Coconut
Fish	All fresh and frozen fish, e.g. cod, plaice, herring, mackerel Tinned fish in brine or tomato sauce, e.g. sardines, tuna	Fish fried in suitable oil Fish fingers or fish cakes (grilled)	Prawns, lobster, crab, oysters, molluscs, winkles Fish tinned in oil (drained)	Fish roe, taramasalata Fried scampi
Meat	Chicken, turkey (without skin) Veal Rabbit Game Soya protein meat substitute Very lean red meat	Lean beef, pork, lamb, ham and gammon Very lean minced meat	Liver, kidney, tripe, sweetbreads Grilled back bacon Duck (without skin) Low-fat pâté	Sausages, luncheon meats, corned beef, pâté, salami, streaky bacon, burgers, goose, meat pies and sausage rolls, pasties, Scotch eggs Visible fat on meat Crackling, chicken skin
Egg and dairy foods	Skimmed milk, soya milk, powdered skimmed milk Cottage cheese Low-fat curd cheese Low-fat yoghurt. Egg white Low-fat fromage frais	Semi-skimmed milk No more than three whole eggs per week including those in baked items, e.g. cakes, quiche, flans	Medium-fat cheeses, e.g. Edam, Camembert, Gouda, Brie, cheese spreads Half-fat cheeses labelled 'low fat' Sweetened condensed skimmed milk	Whole milk and cream Full-fat yoghurt Cheese, e.g. Stilton, Cheddar, cream cheese Evaporated or condensed milk

(Continued p. 160)

Table 11.2 (*Continued*)

Food type	Eat regularly	Eat in moderation occasionally	Eat in moderation special treats	Avoid eating
				Imitation cream Excess eggs, i.e. more than four per week
Fats	Small amounts only—see next column Fat substitute	Margarine and shortenings *labelled 'high in polyunsaturates' or 'mono-unsaturates'* Corn oil, sunflower oil, soya oil, safflower oil, grapeseed oil, olive oil, peanut (ground nut) oil Reduced-fat and low-fat spreads		All margarines, shortenings and oils *not labelled 'high in polyunsaturates' or 'mono-unsaturates'* Butter, lard, suet and dripping Vegetable oil or margarine of unknown origin All spreads not labelled 'low fat'
Prepared foods	Jelly (low sugar) Sorbet Fat-free homemade soups	Pastry, puddings, cakes, biscuits, sauces, etc. made with wholemeal flour and fat or oil as above Low-fat ready-prepared meals	Packet soups Non-dairy ice cream Custard mix made with water or skimmed milk	Pastries, puddings, cakes and sauces made with whole milk and fat or oil as above Suet dumplings or puddings Cream soups
Sweets, preserves, jams and spreads	Marmite, Bovril, chutneys and pickles Sugar-free artificial sweeteners Low-fat jam and marmalade	Fish and meat pastes Peanut butter Jam, marmalade, honey Low-fat soft cheese Low-fat spreads	Boiled sweets, fruit pastilles and jellies	Chocolate spreads Chocolates, toffees, fudge, butterscotch, carob chocolate Coconut bars
Drinks	Freshly made tea, coffee (not too many, not too strong!), mineral water, fruit juice (unsweetened)	Alcohol	Sweetened drinks Squashes, fruit juice (sweetened) Malted milk or hot chocolate drinks made with skimmed milk	Whole milk drinks Cream-based liqueurs Coffee whitener
Sauces and dressings	Herbs, spices, Tabasco, Worcestershire sauce, soy sauce, lemon juice Garlic, pepper	Homemade salad dressings and mayonnaise made with suitable oils as above	'Low-fat' or 'low-calorie' mayonnaise and dressings Parmesan cheese	Ordinary or cream dressings and mayonnaise

Note: If you are overweight, foods high in sugar should be avoided and intake of suitable fats and oils strictly limited.
1. Eat regularly — Choose from this group daily.
2. Eat in moderation — Occasionally, moderate amounts 2–3 times per week. Special treats, moderate amounts once a week or less.
Source: Family Heart Association.

intake. Recently, the Intersalt study demonstrated that populations with high sodium excretion rates are likely to have higher than average systolic blood pressures, and that sodium excretion rates are related to the rise in blood pressure that occurs with age [48]. In a re-analysis of the *cross-sectional* data from Intersalt, the authors have proposed that reductions in sodium intake of 100 mmol day^{-1} would reduce systolic blood pressure by 2.2 mmHg and diastolic blood pressure by 0.1 mmHg [49]. Whilst this approximates to estimates made from meta-analysis of salt restriction studies [50], extrapolations of cross-sectional data should not be taken as evidence that salt restriction leads to blood pressure reductions. In any case, such reductions are small compared to the typical reduction of approximately 12% [51] achieved by antihypertensive drugs.

It is likely that the issue of salt in hypertension will never be resolved, for a longitudinal study to monitor sodium chloride intake and blood pressure prospectively in a sufficiently large population will never be performed [46]. Against this background are reports that salt restriction may lead to elevations in serum cholesterol, impairment in glucose tolerance [52] and increased incidence of MI and total cardiovascular disease [53]. As a further complication, adherence to low-salt diets is very poor, even in well-motivated participants of clinical trials [1,54].

The blood pressure lowering effect of dietary salt restriction alone is of questionable therapeutic value. The magnitude of the reduction in blood pressure is certainly less than that achieved by avoiding excessive alcohol intake [43,55,56]. Salt restriction does lessen the requirement for higher doses of antihypertensive drugs [57]. A realistic target is to reduce sodium chloride intake to 6 g day^{-1} (100 mmol day^{-1}) [58,59] in combination with weight reduction and moderate alcohol intake [60]. Attempts to reduce dietary sodium chloride intake to < 70 mmol l^{-1} are destined to make the patient's life a misery and therefore, are likely to fail [61]. The following measures should be adopted:

- *Avoid processed foods* (Table 11.3) — up to 85% of dietary salt comes from processed foods [62]. Conventional processed foods should be discouraged and versions with the 'no added salt' label encouraged as alternatives [63]. It should be noted that salt is the main source of flavour in processed foods.
- *Avoid adding salt at the table* — ingredients such as fresh fruit, fresh vegetables, herbs and unprocessed condiments improve flavour and curtail the need for salt in cooking.

Other mineral salts

Potassium supplementation has invariably been shown to produce negligible blood pressure reductions [55,64,65] and it is, therefore, not recommended in the treatment of hypertension. Magnesium [55,66] and calcium [67,68]

Table 11.3 Foods with a high sodium content.

Cured meats
Bacon, ham, Parma ham, chorizos, salami
Tinned foods
Meats (corned beef, spam, chopped ham and pork)
Fish (smoked haddock, kippers) and shellfish
Soup, vegetables, tomato juice
Pre-prepared foods
Pizzas, frozen dinners, stews, chilli
Sausages, hamburgers, beefburgers, pies
Meat paste and fish paste
Cheese
Pickles, Bovril, Oxo, Marmite, Bisto, gravy browning
Crisps, pretzels, salted peanuts, savoury snacks, peanut butter, white chocolate, olives

supplementation have not been shown to be beneficial in blood pressure lowering.

Fish and fish oils

A randomized controlled trial has shown that eating fish at least three times per week reduces the incidence of myocardial re-infarction [69]. Data on the possible hypotensive effects of ω-3 marine oils [70–72] are conflicting [73] and there are no sound data at present to recommend their specific use in hypertension or in CHD risk reduction. Indeed, there is some evidence that they may be harmful [74]. On the other hand, supplementation with ω-3 marine oils should be considered in patients with severe hypertriglyceridaemia.

Anti-oxidants

Although popular, the notion that anti-oxidants may be beneficial in CHD [75] has not been substantiated by clinical outcome data. Some prospective observational studies have shown an inverse relationship between high intake of anti-oxidant vitamins and CHD risk [75,76], but randomized trials of beta-carotene and vitamin E supplementation have shown no benefit [77]. An increased risk of cerebral haemorrhage has been associated with vitamin E supplementation [78]. Data on the benefits of vitamin C are inconsistent [76]. The notion that folic acid might protect against CHD by lowering plasma homocysteine levels remains unsubstantiated.

ALCOHOL

Evidence relating to the pressor effects of ethanol has generally been derived from studies of individuals consuming large amounts of ethanol (80 g day^{-1}) [79–82]. In such studies, definitions of 'excessive' alcohol intake have differed

Table 11.4 Advice on alcohol for patients.

Excessive drinking
Raises blood pressure and increases the chances of developing a stroke
Increases the chances of developing liver damage, including cirrhosis, and cancers of the throat and mouth
Reduces fertility and impairs development of the baby in the womb

Moderate drinking
Is likely to make you live longer than those who don't drink at all
Increases the 'good' blood cholesterol
Between 1 and 2 units of alcohol per day on a regular basis provides the maximum advantage on health
1 or 2 units once or twice a week is safe for women who are trying to become pregnant or at any stage of pregnancy
Binge drinking confers little benefit
The type of drink, for example, red wine, does not protect you more than other drinks

Total abstinence is recommended if you have
Uncontrolled hypertension
Heart failure or asymptomatic ventricular dysfunction
Cardiac arrhythmias
Hypertriglyceridaemia

widely (from 18 g to 200 g). As a result, these studies may not be relevant to clinical practice. There is no doubt that abstinence in alcoholic individuals reduces blood pressure [80]. There is, however, considerable variation in the susceptibility to the pressor effects of ethanol between individuals [83]. The effects of alcohol on aspects other than blood pressure need to be considered. Levels above 40 g day^{-1}, however, are associated with an increased risk of haemorrhagic stroke. Heavy drinkers (more than six drinks per day) also have a higher risk of sudden death [84].

On the other hand, numerous studies have shown that mild-to-moderate alcohol drinking in both men and women is cardioprotective [85–87]. This relationship is J-shaped [88], with the lowest mortality occurring in individuals consuming one or two drinks per day [89], followed by teetotallers and occasional drinkers and then by those consuming more than three drinks per day. The cardiovascular benefits are seen in individuals who consume up to 40–50 g day^{-1} of ethanol [90]. The mechanism for the cardioprotection afforded by alcohol remains elusive. Up to 50% of the protective effect on CHD may be related to increases in HDL-cholesterol [91–93], an effect that is apparent in individuals consuming moderate amounts [94]. Other factors such as lowering of plasma fibrinogen, reduced platelet aggregation, increased fibrinolysis and increased insulin sensitivity may also be involved.

The advice for hypertensive patients (Table 11.4) should be to keep alcohol intake certainly < 40 g day^{-1} and, ideally, between 1 and 2 units of alcohol

Table 11.5 Units of alcohol in usual drinks*.

	Alcohol By Volume (ABV) (%)	25 ml measure ('single')	50 ml measure ('double')	125 ml ('glass')	330 ml bottle	1 pint or 440 ml can	500 ml can	75 cl bottle
Beer, lager or cider								
Standard strength	4–5				1.5	2	2–2.5	3–3.8
'Strong'	8–9				2.5–3	3.5–4	4–4.5	6–6.8
'Low' alcohol	1.2				0.4	0.5	0.6	1
Wine	9–10			1–1.3				7–7.5
	11–12			1.5				8–9
Sherry, Port, Madeira, Vermouth	15–17.5		1					11–13
'Alco-pops'	4–6				1.5–2			
	13.5				4.5			
Spirit (whisky, gin, vodka)	40	1	2					30

*Units of alcohol = [volume of drink in ml × Alcohol By Volume (ABV) %]/1000. 1 unit = 8 g ethanol = 10 ml by volume of pure ethanol [95].

per day on a regular basis i.e. 10–30 g of ethanol per day for men and 10–20 g per day for women. It is often helpful for patients to quantify what they drink (Table 11.5). One should be realistic in advising hypertensive patients that reducing alcohol consumption by 80% may reduce systolic blood pressure by 5 mmHg and diastolic blood pressure by 3 mmHg.

> 1 unit = 8 g ethanol [95] = 10 ml by volume of pure ethanol
> Units of alcohol = (volume of drink × Alcohol By Volume %)/1000
> 1 unit = $^1/_2$ pint of standard strength beer or cider
>   *or* 1 glass of wine
>   *or* 1 single measure of spirit or fortified wine, such as sherry

Although some studies have suggested that red wine might be particularly protective [96,97], no evidence-based recommendations can be made on preferences of one type of alcoholic beverage over another. The reasons as to why Mediterranean countries have a low incidence of CHD remain unclear. Factors other than alcohol, including the use of olive oil, natural anti-oxidants and genetic factors are likely to play a role.

Alcoholic cardiomyopathy occurs in patients with an alcohol intake of > 80 g day[-1] for at least 10 years, or a cumulative lifetime intake of 250 kg of ethanol [98]. The ECG frequently shows non-specific ST and T wave abnormalities [99]. Atrial fibrillation is the commonest presenting arrhythmia, but sinus tachycardia and ventricular arrhythmias also occur. Early detection of alcoholic cardiomyopathy [100] is important, as disturbances of myocardial function may be reversible [101].

In conclusion, the beneficial effects of alcohol are probably limited to up to three drinks per day. Above this, there is an increased risk of developing hypertension in susceptible individuals. It is unknown whether reducing alcohol intake long term lowers blood pressure. Recommendations to lower alcohol intake below two drinks per day are unjustified in most circumstances.

Summary of lifestyle modifications for all individuals, hypertensive or normotensive

- Stop smoking
- Lose weight to keep BMI between 20 and 25 kg m^{-2}. Aim to lose 0.5–1 kg week^{-1} (not more) by avoiding fatty foods, sugar and alcohol. Crash diets do not help in the long term
- Limit alcohol intake to 10–30 g of ethanol per day for men and 10–20 g per day for women
- Walk briskly for $\approx$ 45 min per day on most days of the week
- Keep to a good diet for reducing coronary risk:
  - Avoid processed foods
  - Keep daily salt (sodium chloride) intake < 6 g day^{-1} by*:
    Avoiding processed foods and other salty foods
    Avoiding adding salt at the table
  - Keep to a low daily total and saturated fat intake
  - Eat fresh fruit and vegetables with every meal
  - Eat foods containing soluble fibre at least once a day
  - Eat fish at least three times a week

---

*Whether salt intake should be reduced in normotensive patients is a contentious issue that has not been adequately assessed.

References

1   Langford HG, Davis BR, Blaufox D *et al.* Effect of drug and diet treatment of mild hypertension on diastolic blood pressure. *Hypertension* 1991; 17: 210–217.

2   Bonita R, Scragg S, Stewart A, Jackson J, Beaglehole R. Cigarette smoking and the risk of premature stroke in men and women. *BMJ* 1986; 293: 6–8.

3   Asmar RG, Girerd XJ, Brahimi M *et al.* Ambulatory blood pressure measurement, smoking and abnormalities of glucose and lipid metabolism in essential hypertension. *J Hum Hypertens* 1992; 10: 181–187.

4   Groppelli A, Giorgi DMA, Omboni S *et al.* Persistent blood pressure increase induced by heavy smoking. *J Hypertens* 1992; 10: 495–499.

5   Doll R, Peto R. Mortality in relation to smoking: 20 years' observation on male British doctors. *BMJ* 1976; 2: 1525–1536.

6   Kawachi I, Colditz GA, Stampfer MJ *et al.* Smoking cessation in relation to total mortality rates in women. A prospective cohort study. *Ann Intern Med* 1993; 119: 992–1000.

7   Hermanson B, Omenn GS, Kronmal RA, Gersh BJ and participants in the coronary artery surgery study. Beneficial six-year outcome of smoking cessation in older men and women with coronary artery disease. Results from the CASS registry. *N Engl J Med* 1988; 319: 1365–1369.

8   Kottke TE, Batiska RN, Fries GH. Attributes of successful smoking cessation interventions in medical practice: a meta-analysis of 39 controlled trials. *JAMA* 1988; 259: 2882–2889.

9   ICRF General Practice Research Group. Randomized trial of nicotine patches in general practice: results at one year. *BMJ* 1994; 308: 1476–1477.

10 Working Group for Study of Transdermal Nicotine Patches in Patients with Coronary Heart Disease. Nicotine replacement for patients with coronary heart disease. *Arch Intern Med* 1994; 154: 989–995.

11 Rissanen AM, Heliovaara M, Knekt P *et al.* Determinants of weight gain and overweight in adult Finns. *Eur J Clin Nutr* 1991; 45: 419–430.

12 Thorne MC, Wing AL, Paffenbarger RS Jr. Chronic disease in former college students. VII. Early precursors in nonfatal coronary heart disease. *Am J Epidemiol* 1968; 87: 520–529.

13 Blair SN, Goodyear NN, Gibbons LW *et al.* Physical fitness and incidence of hypertension in healthy normotensive men and women. *JAMA* 1984; 252: 487–490.

14 Ekelund LG, Haskell WL, Johnson JL *et al.* Physical fitness as a predictor of cardiovascular mortality in asymptomatic North American men. The Lipid Research Clinics mortality follow-up study. *N Engl J Med* 1988; 319: 1379–1384.

15 Jennings GL, Deakin G, Korner P *et al.* What is the dose–response relationship between exercise training and blood pressure? *Ann Med* 1991; 23: 313–318.

16 Foster WR, Burton BT. National Institutes of Health consensus conference: health implications of obesity. *Ann Intern Med* 1985; 103: 977–1077.

17 Van Itallie TB, Kral JG. The dilemma of morbid obesity. *JAMA* 1981; 246: 999–1003.

18 Hubert HB, Feinleib M, McNamara PM *et al.* Obesity as an independent risk factor for cardiovascular disease: a 26-year follow-up of participants in the Framingham Heart Study. *Circulation* 1983; 67: 968–977.

19 Rhoads GG, Kagan A. The relation of coronary disease, stroke, and mortality to weight in youth and middle age. *Lancet* 1983; 1: 492–495.

20 Dietz WH. Childhood obesity: susceptibility, cause, and management. *J Pediatr* 1983; 103: 676–686.

21 Stunkard AJ. Conservative treatments for obesity. *Am J Clin Nutr* 1987; 45: 1142–1154.

22 NIH Technology Assessment Conference Panel. Methods for voluntary weight loss and control. Technology Assessment Conference Statement. *Ann Intern Med* 1993; 119: 764–770.

23 Wadden TA. Treatment of obesity by moderate and severe caloric restriction: results of clinical research trials. *Ann Intern Med* 1993; 119: 688–693.

24 Blair SN. Evidence for success of exercise in weight loss and control. *Ann Intern Med* 1993; 119: 702–706.

25 Pi-Sunyer FX. Medical hazards of obesity. *Ann Intern Med* 1993; 119: 655–660.

26 Manson JE, Colditz GA, Stampfer MJ *et al.* A prospective study of obesity and risk of coronary heart disease in women. *N Engl J Med* 1990; 322: 882–889.

27   Ohlson LO, Larsson B, Svardsudd K *et al.* The influence of body fat distribution on the incidence of diabetes mellitus: 13.5 years of follow-up of the participants in the study of men born in 1913. *Diabetes* 1985; 34: 1055–1058.

28   Smoak CG, Burke GL, Webber LS, Harsha DW, Srinivasan SR, Berenson GS. Relation of obesity to clustering of cardiovascular disease risk factors in children and young adults: the Bogalusa heart study. *Am J Epidemiol* 1987; 125: 364–372.

29   Aristimuno GG, Foster TA, Voors AW *et al.* Influence of persistent obesity in children on cardiovascular risk factors: the Bogalusa Heart Study. *Circulation* 1984; 69: 895–904.

30   Wannamethee G, Shaper AG. Weight change in middle-aged British men: implications for health. *Eur J Clin Nutr* 1990; 44: 133–142.

31   Bray GA. Obesity: basic considerations and clinical approaches. *Dis Month* 1989; 35: 449–537.

32   Van Itallie TB. Health implications of overweight and obesity in the United States. *Ann Intern Med* 1985; 103: 983–988.

33   Corr LA, Oliver MF. The low fat/low cholesterol diet is ineffective. *Eur Heart J* 1997; 18: 18–22.

34   Katzel LI, Bleecher ER, Colman EG, Rogus EM, Sorkin JD, Goldberg AP. Effects of weight loss vs aerobic exercise training on risk factors for coronary disease in healthy, obese, middle-aged and older men. A randomized controlled trial. *JAMA* 1996; 274: 1915–1921.

35   Ramsay LE, Yeo WW, Jackson PR. Dietary reduction of serum cholesterol concentration: time to think again. *BMJ* 1996; 303: 953–957.

36   Family Heart Study Group. Randomized controlled trial evaluating cardiovascular screening and intervention in general practice; principal results of British family heart study. *BMJ* 1994; 308: 313–320.

37   Imperial Cancer Research Fund OXCHECK Study Group. Effectiveness of health checks conducted by nurses in primary care: final results of the OXCHECK Study. *BMJ* 1995; 310: 1099–1104.

38   Tang JL, Armitage JM, Lancaster T, Silagy CA, Fowler GH, Neil HAW. Systematic review of dietary intervention trials to lower blood cholesterol in free-living subjects. *BMJ* 1998; 316: 1213–1219.

39   Expert Panel of Detection, Evaluation and Treatment of High Blood Cholesterol in Adults. Summary of the second report of the National Cholesterol Education Program (NCEP) Expert Panel on detection, evaluation, and treatment of high blood cholesterol in adults (Acute Treatment Panel II). *JAMA* 1993; 269: 3015–3023.

40   Hunninghake DB, Stein EA, Dujovne CA *et al.* The efficacy of intensive dietary therapy alone or combined with lovastatin in outpatients with hypercholesterolemia. *N Engl J Med* 1993; 328: 1213–1219.

41   Simpson FO. Salt and hypertension: a sceptical review of the evidence. *Clin Sci* 1979; 57 (Suppl.): 463–469.

42   Nicholls MG. Reduction of dietary sodium in Western Society: benefit or risk? *Hypertension* 1984; 6: 795–801.

43   Swales JD. Salt saga continued: salt has only small importance in hypertension. *BMJ* 1988; 297: 307–308.

44   Muntzel M, Drüeke T. A comprehensive review of the salt and blood pressure relationship. *Am J Hypertens* 1992; 5 (Suppl.): 1–42.

45   Kurtz TW, Al-Bander HA, Morris RC. 'Salt-sensitive' hypertension in men: is the sodium ion alone important? *N Engl J Med* 1987; 317: 1043–1048.

46   Thelle DS. Salt and blood pressure revisited. *BMJ* 1996; 312: 1240–1241.

47 Denton D, Weisinger R, Mundy NI *et al*. The effect of increased salt intake on blood pressure of chimpanzees. *Nature Med* 1995; 1: 1009–1016.

48 Intersalt Cooperative Research Group. Intersalt: an international study of electrolyte excretion and blood pressure. Results for 24 hour urinary sodium and potassium. *BMJ* 1988; 297: 319–328.

49 Elliot P, Stamler J, Nichols R *et al*. Intersalt revisited: further analyses of 24 hour sodium excretion and blood pressure within and across populations. *BMJ* 1996; 312: 1249–1253.

50 Elliot P. Observational studies of salt and blood pressure. *Hypertension* 1991; 17 (Suppl. 1): 3–8.

51 Lewis CE, Grandits GA, Flack J *et al*. Efficacy and tolerance of antihypertensive treatment in men and women with stage I diastolic hypertension: results of the Treatment of Mild Hypertension Study. *Arch Intern Med* 1996; 156: 377–385.

52 Iwaoka T, Umeda T, Inoue J *et al*. Dietary NaCl restriction deteriorates glucose tolerance in hypertensive patients with impairment of glucose tolerance. *Am J Hypertens* 1994; 7: 460–463.

53 Alderman MH, Cohen H, Madhaven S. Low urinary sodium and increased myocardial infarction and total cardiovascular disease among treated hypertensives. *J Hypertens* 1992; 10 (Suppl. 4): 137.

54 Hypertension Prevention Trial Research Group. The Hypertension Prevention Trial: three-year effects of dietary changes on blood pressure. *Arch Intern Med* 1990; 150: 153–162.

55 Ramsay LE. Dietary aspects of prevention and treatment of hypertension. *Curr Opin Cardiol* 1987; 2: 758–763.

56 Alderman MH, Lamport B. Moderate sodium restriction: do the benefits justify the hazards? *Am J Hypertens* 1990; 3: 499–504.

57 World Hypertension League. Non-pharmacological interventions as an adjunct to the pharmacological treatment of hypertension: a statement by WHL. *J Hum Hypertens* 1993; 7: 159–164.

58 US Department of Health and Human Services. Health People 2000: National health promotion and disease prevention objectives (summary report). Washington: Government Printing Office, 1991 (DHHS Publication No. (PHS) 91-50213).

59 The National Nutrition Council. Dietary recommendations. Oslo: NNC, 1989.

60 Berglund A, Andersson OK, Gerglund G, Fagerberg B. Antihypertensive effect of diet compared to drug treatment in obese men with mild hypertension. *BMJ* 1989; 299: 480–485.

61 Wassertheil-Smoller S, Oberman A, Blaufox MD *et al*. The Trial of Antihypertensive Interventions and Management (TAIM) Study. Final results with regard to blood pressure, cardiovascular risk, and quality of life. *Am J Hypertens* 1992; 5: 37–44.

62 Gregory J, Forster K, Tyler H, Wiseman M. *The Dietary and Nutritional Survey of British Adults*. London: HMSO, 1990.

63 Godlee F. The food industry fights for salt. *BMJ* 1996; 312: 1239–1240.

64 Matlou SM, Isles CG, Higgs A *et al*. Potassium supplementation in blacks with mild to moderate essential hypertension. *J Hypertens* 1986; 4: 61–65.

65 Beilin LJ. Environmental and dietary aspects of primary hypertension. In: Robertson J, ed. *Handbook of Clinical Hypertension*. Amsterdam: Elsevier, 1992: 95–140.

66 Cappuccio FP, Markandu ND, Beynon GW *et al*. Lack of effect of oral magnesium on high blood pressure: a double blind study. *BMJ* 1985; 291: 235–238.

67 Zoccali C, Mallami F, Delfino D *et al*. Long-term oral calcium supplementation in hypertension: a double-blind, randomized, cross-over study. *J Hypertens* 1986; 4 (Suppl. 6): 676–678.

68 Bloomfield RL, Young LD, Zurek G *et al*. Effects of oral calcium carbonate in subjects with mildly elevated arterial pressure. *J Hypertens* 1986; 4 (Suppl. 5): 351–354.

69 Burr ML, Fehily AM, Gilbert JF *et al*. Effects of changes in fat, fish and fibre intakes on death and myocardial reinfarction: diet and reinfarction trial (DART). *Lancet* 1989; ii: 757–761.

70 Bonna KU, Straume B, Gram IT, Thelle D. Effect of eicosapentaenoic and docosa-hexaenoic acids on blood pressure in hypertension. *N Engl J Med* 1990; 322: 795–801.

71 Mortensen JZ, Schmidt EB, Nielsen AH, Dyerberg J. The effects of n-6 and n-3 polyunsaturated fatty acids on hemostasis, blood lipids and blood pressure. *Thromb Haemost* 1983; 50: 543–546.

72 Knapp HR, Fitzgerald GA. The antihypertensive effects of fish oil: a controlled study of polyunsaturated fatty acid supplements in essential hypertension. *N Engl J Med* 1989; 320: 1037–1043.

73 Hypertension Prevention Collaborative Research Group. The effects of non-pharmacological interventions on blood pressure of persons with high normal levels. *JAMA* 1992; 267: 1212–1220.

74 Daviglus ML, Stamler J, Greenland P, Dyer AR, Liu K. Fish consumption and risk of coronary heart disease. What does the evidence show? *Eur Heart J* 1997; 18: 1841–1842.

75 Steinberg D, Parthasarathy S, Carew TE, Khoo JC, Witztum JL. Beyond cholesterol: modifications of low-density lipoprotein that increase its atherogenicity. *N Engl J Med* 1989; 320: 915–924.

76 Enstrom JE, Kanim LE, Klein MA. Vitamin C and mortality among a sample of the United States population. *Epidemiology* 1992; 3: 194–202.

77 The Alpha-Tocopherol Beta Carotene Cancer Prevention Study Group. The effect of vitamin E and beta carotene on the incidence of lung cancer and other cancers in male smokers. *N Engl J Med* 1994; 330: 1029–1035.

78 Hennekens CH, Buring JE, Peto R. Anti-oxidant vitamins — benefits not yet proved. *N Engl J Med* 1994; 330: 1080–1081.

79 Saunders JB, Beevers DG, Paton A. Alcohol-induced hypertension. *Lancet* 1981; ii: 653–656.

80 Potter JF, Beevers DG. Pressor effects of alcohol in hypertension. *Lancet* 1984; i: 119–122.

81 Saunders JB, Beevers DG, Patin A. Factors influencing blood pressure in chronic alcoholics. *Clin Sci* 1979; 57: 295s–298s.

82 Wrenn KD, Slovis CM, Minion GE *et al*. The syndrome of alcoholic ketoacidosis. *Am J Med* 1991; 91: 119–128.

83 Vandongen R, Puddey IB. Alcohol intake and blood pressure. In: Swales J, ed. *Textbook of Hypertension*. Oxford: Blackwell Scientific Publications, 1994: 567–575.

84 Wannamethee G, Shaper AG. Alcohol and sudden cardiac death. *Br Heart J* 1992; 68: 443–448.

85 Friedman HS. Cardiovascular effects of ethanol. In: Lieber C, ed. *Medical and Nutritional Complications of Alcoholism: Mechanisms and Management*. New York: Plenum, 1977: 359–401.

86 Rimm EB, Giovannucci EL, Willet WC *et al*. Prospective study of alcohol consumption and risk of coronary heart disease in men. *Lancet* 1991; 338: 464–468.

87 Stamfer MJ, Colditz GA, Willet WC, Speizer FE, Hennekens CH. A prospective study of moderate alcohol consumption and the risk of coronary heart disease and stroke in women. *N Engl J Med* 1988; 319: 267–273.

88 Klatsky AL, Armstrong MA, Friedman GD. Alcohol and mortality. *Ann Intern Med* 1992; 117: 646–654.

89   McGinnis JM, Foege WH. Actual causes of death in the United States. *JAMA* 1993; 270: 2207–2212.

90   Yano K, Rhoads GG, Kagan A. Coffee, alcohol and risk of coronary heart disease among Japanese men living in Hawaii. *N Engl J Med* 1977; 297: 405–409.

91   Masarei JRL, Puddey IB, Rouse IL, Lynch WJ, Vandongen R, Beilin LJ. Effects of alcohol consumption on serum lipoprotein-lipid and apolipoprotein concentrations: results from an intervention study in healthy subjects. *Atherosclerosis* 1986; 60: 79–87.

92   Gordon T, Ernst N, Fisher M, Rifkind BM. Alcohol and high-density lipoprotein cholesterol. *Circulation* 1981; 64 (Suppl. III): III-57–III-63.

93   Suh I, Shaten BJ, Cutler JA, Kuller LJH. Research Group for the Multiple Risk Factor Intervention Trial. Alcohol use and mortality from coronary heart disease: the role of high-density lipoprotein cholesterol. *Ann Intern Med* 1992; 116: 881–887.

94   Haskell WL, Camargo C Jr, Williams PT *et al*. The effect of cessation and resumption of moderate alcohol intake on serum high-density-lipoprotein subfractions: a controlled study. *N Engl J Med* 1984; 310: 805–810.

95   Royal College of Physicians, Royal College of Psychiatrists and Royal College of General Practitioners. *Alcohol and the Heart in Perspective. Sensible Limits Reaffirmed*. London: Chameleon Press, 1995.

96   Sharp D. Coronary disease: when wine is red. *Lancet* 1993; 341: 27–28.

97   Frankel EN, Kanner J, German JB *et al*. Inhibition of human low-density lipoprotein by phenolic substances in red wine. *Lancet* 1993; 341: 454–457.

98   Richardson PJ, Wodak AA. Alcohol-induced heart muscle disease. In: Symons C, Evans T, Mitchell A, eds. *Specific Heart Muscle Disease*. Bristol: Wright, PSG, 1983: 99–122.

99   McCall D. Alcohol and the cardiovascular system. *Curr Probl Cardiol* 1987; 12: 353–414.

100   Kupari M, Koskinen P, Suokas A, Ventila M. Left ventricular filling impairment in asymptomatic chronic alcoholics. *Am J Cardiol* 1990; 66: 1473–1477.

101   Auffermann W, Wu ST, Wikman-Coffelt J, Parmley WW. Cardiac function and metabolism after chronic alcohol consumption: adaptation, reversibility and effects of verapamil. *Am Heart J* 1991; 122: 122–126.

12: Pharmacological Treatment

The ultimate aim of antihypertensive treatment is to prevent end-organ damage, overt clinical disease and death. In order to achieve this within the constraints of a public heath system, the ideal antihypertensive agent should:
- Provide effective 24-h control of both systolic and diastolic blood pressures.
- Minimize increased blood pressure variability and the early morning blood pressure surge. A slow onset and a long duration of action are preferable. These properties should be intrinsic to the drug, rather than to slow release formulations.
- Retard the progression or reverse end-organ damage, such as LVH and dysfunction, cardiac dysrhythmias and renal failure.
- Have neutral or favourable effects on disturbances that are *related* to hypertension, such as dyslipidaemia, left ventricular hypertrophy and cardiac arrhythmias, and renal impairment.
- Not exacerbate comorbid conditions that are *unrelated* to hypertension, such as bronchoconstriction.
- Not produce symptomatic side-effects.
- Not produce clinical and biochemical side-effects that require additional clinical supervision.
- Not reduce the patient's quality of life.
- Be simple to comply with.
- Be competitively priced.

No antihypertensive drug satisfies all the above criteria. Despite the availability of a large armamentarium of antihypertensive drugs, few drugs are clearly superior to others on the basis of antihypertensive efficacy and tolerability [1]. Whilst most of the drugs currently available have similar antihypertensive effects, some have added qualities that make them particularly suitable for individual patients. In choosing the appropriate drug, the clinician must start from the patient rather than from the drug. One should then choose the drug class and then, an individual drug within the class (Fig. 12.1).

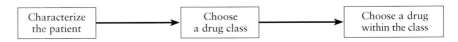

Figure 12.1 Steps in the choice of antihypertensive drugs.

THIAZIDE DIURETICS

Effects

Thiazide diuretics, whose mechanism of action is shown in Fig. 12.2, are effective at lowering blood pressure. They have, in combination with β-blockers, been shown to prevent mortality from stroke and CHD in non-diabetic patients with *mild-to-moderate* essential hypertension [2–4]. It

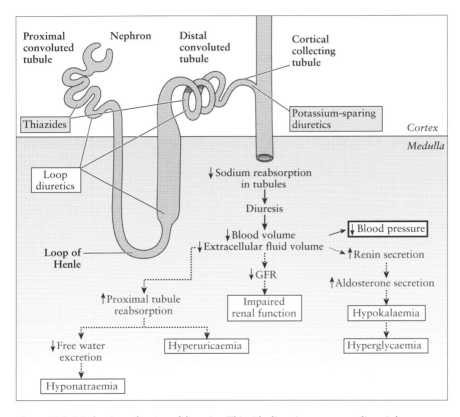

Figure 12.2 Mechanism of action of diuretics. Thiazide diuretics promote a diuresis by interfering with the transport of sodium chloride from the lumen of the distal convoluted tubule to the cells that line the tubules. The initial hypotensive effect results from natriuresis, a reduction in plasma and extracellular fluid volume, and a reduction in cardiac output. Vasodilator effects are not direct but rather, secondary to volume depletion. During prolonged treatment, renal sodium excretion parallels dietary sodium intake, plasma volume and cardiac output tend to normalize, and the subsequent reduction in peripheral resistance sustains the chronic hypotensive effect. In addition to their natriuretic effect, thiazides also promote potassium loss. This is caused by their actions on the renal tubule as well as by their additional, inhibitory effect on carbonic anhydrase and their capacity to cause elevations in circulating aldosterone. Reductions in the clearance of uric acid lead to hyperuricaemia. Through mechanisms which remain unclear, thiazides at high doses worsen glucose tolerance. GFR, glomerular filtration rate.

should be noted that in the large hypertension trials, diuretic therapy has often been combined with other agents [5] and the doubt still remains as to whether diuretic *monotherapy* can achieve reductions in mortality [6].

Although moderate salt restriction appears to enhance the hypotensive effect of thiazides, this is seldom clinically significant. Thiazide diuretics are usually not effective when there is increased sodium and water retention such as in heart failure, or when the glomerular filtration rate is below 30 ml min^{-1} (plasma creatinine > 150 µmol l^{-1}).

The modified thiazide indapamide is an effective antihypertensive agent which has negligible effects on serum lipids or glucose levels at a dose of 1.25–2.5 mg o.d. Reductions in serum potassium are dose related, but negligible at low doses (1.25 mg o.d.: 0.3 mEq l^{-1}; 10 mg o.d.: 0.8 mEq l^{-1}) [7].

Cautions and adverse effects

Electrolyte disturbances. Hypokalaemia is of particular concern in patients with CHD and those taking digoxin, in whom it may precipitate serious arrhythmias. The risk of hypokalaemia is more dependent on duration of action than on potency. It is more common with the longer acting chlorthalidone, even at low doses of 15–30 mg. Hypokalaemia is dose dependent: with bendrofluazide at a dose of 10 mg, up to 50% of hypertensive patients have a serum potassium < 3.5 mmol l^{-1}. It is also more common in women than in men, and if daily dosages are divided. If hypokalaemia develops, we recommend changing to a different class of antihypertensive agent. Hyponatraemia, hypomagnesaemia and hypochloraemic alkalosis can also occur.

Impotence. The incidence of impotence has probably been overestimated in single-blind trials using high-dose regimens, in which concurrent treatment with other drugs may have also contributed. Thiazide diuretics are, however, occasionally responsible for impotence, which is reversible on withdrawal of the drug.

Gout and hyperuricaemia. Thiazide diuretics cause hyperuricaemia [8] by increasing the tubular reabsorption of uric acid. Whilst thiazides should be avoided in patients with a history of gout, hyperuricaemia without previous attacks of gout or urate nephrolithiasis should not preclude prescription of a thiazide diuretic. The risk of gout is increased at thiazide doses of hydrochlorothiazide 25 mg day^{-1} (or equivalents), but not at lower doses [9].

Lipid and carbohydrate metabolism. Thiazide diuretics induce transient elevations in total plasma cholesterol, triglycerides and LDL-cholesterol at high doses [10], but not at low doses [11] (Table 12.1). The TOMH study

[12] and the EWPHE trial [13] detected no changes in total cholesterol between thiazide-treated and placebo-controlled groups. Some dose-related changes in total cholesterol may be observed in patients who have low cholesterol levels. Thiazide-related elevations in cholesterol do not persist beyond the first year of treatment. An elevated plasma cholesterol is *not* a contra-indication to the use of thiazide diuretics.

Table 12.1 Effects of bendrofluazide 2.5 mg o.d. on blood pressure and biochemical parameters.

Systolic blood pressure (mmHg)	↓ 11.5*
Diastolic blood pressure (mmHg)	↓ 7.3*
Potassium (mmol l^{-1})	↓ 0.29*
Uric acid (μmol l^{-1})	↑ 34*
Glucose (mmol l^{-1})	↑ 0.22
Cholesterol (mmol l^{-1})†	↑ 0.06
Creatinine (mol l^{-1})	↑ 5.2*

*$P < 0.05$ compared to placebo. Adapted from [15].
†Note that according to a recent meta-analysis [17], a 1% reduction in total cholesterol with lipid-lowering treatment, equivalent to a mean reduction of 0.06 mmol l^{-1} in a population with a mean cholesterol level of 6.0 mmol l^{-1}, translates to a 1% reduction in all-cause mortality.

Other rare side-effects. Neutropenia and thrombocytopenia; skin rashes; blood dyscrasias; nephritis; pneumonitis; pancreatitis; cholestatic jaundice; and acute cholecystitis.

Interactions

Thiazide-induced hypokalaemia can predispose to ventricular arrhythmias in patients taking digoxin or drugs that prolong the Q–T interval. Non-steroidal anti-inflammatory drugs reduce the antihypertensive actions of thiazides. Thiazides reduce renal clearance and increase the plasma levels of lithium.

Absolute contra-indications

Hypercalcaemia.

Choice

Bendrofluazide is superior to hydrochlorothiazide and chlorthalidone in providing effective 24-h control of blood pressure whilst minimizing electrolyte and metabolic disturbances.

Doses

Whether thiazides are adequately antihypertensive at the low doses required to minimize their metabolic side-effects is open to debate [14]. Some argue that because with thiazides the dose–blood pressure response curve is relatively flat [15], high doses achieve little therapeutic advantage over lower doses. Others [14] note that low-dose diuretics are effective in only *mild* hypertension (as in the TOMH study [12]) and that high, metabolically adverse doses are needed in patients with higher blood pressure levels.

On balance, we recommend that thiazides should be used at low doses and not titrated. Higher (bendrofluazide > 2.5 mg, hydrochlorothiazide 50 mg o.d.) do not produce a better antihypertensive effect and lead to an increased frequency of metabolic disturbances and cardiac arrhythmias [16]. The optimal doses which, in mild hypertension, ensure a satisfactory 24-h antihypertensive effect whilst minimizing metabolic disturbances are:

Preference

Bendrofluazide 2.5 mg o.d.
Chlorthalidone 15 mg o.d.
Hydrochlorothiazide 12.5 mg o.d. (hydrochlorothiazide 6.25 mg o.d. may also be effective)

Follow-up

There is no need to dose-titrate thiazide diuretics. The maximum antihypertensive effect with thiazides occurs between 6 and 12 weeks [18]. Because of metabolic side-effects (Table 12.1), electrolytes should be checked at 3–4 weeks after starting treatment. Discontinuation of treatment should be considered if the plasma potassium falls to ≤ 3.4 mmol l^{-1}, particularly in patients with heart disease or who are otherwise predisposed to ventricular arrhythmias [19]. As with all other antihypertensive drugs, $\approx 10\%$ of patients discontinue diuretic therapy. The reason for discontinuation is often light-headedness on standing up, without there being a demonstrable postural blood pressure drop. Treatment should be discontinued if the patient develops gout or serious side-effects (skin rashes, blood dyscrasias, nephritis, pneumonitis, pancreatitis, cholestatic jaundice and acute cholecystitis). Withdrawal of long-term diuretic therapy in elderly patients can precipitate heart failure and therefore, careful monitoring is advised during the initial 4 weeks of withdrawal [20].

β-ADRENOCEPTOR BLOCKERS

Effects

β-Blockers have, in combination with thiazide diuretics, been shown to reduce morbidity from stroke and CHD in non-diabetic hypertensive patients. As

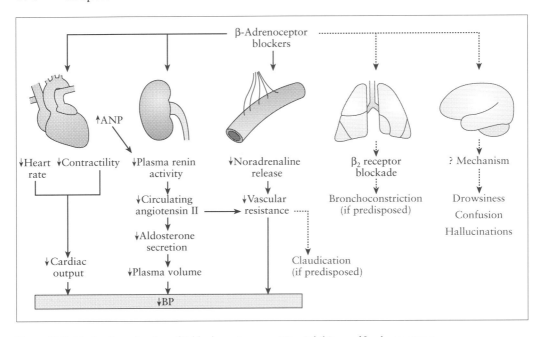

Figure 12.3 Mechanism of action of β-blockers. As competitive inhibitors of β-adrenoceptors, their antihypertensive effects are principally mediated by inhibition of sympathetic supply to the sinoatrial node, which reduces heart rate and cardiac output. Other actions include alterations in baroreceptor reflex sensitivity, a reduction in myocardial contractility, alterations in plasma renin activity and inhibition of peripheral sympathetic tone. Through central mechanims which remain elusive, β-blockers cause drowsiness, confusion and hallucinations. This is most often seen with the lipid-soluble β-blockers. ANP, atrial natriuretic peptide.

for thiazide diuretics, β-blockers have invariably been combined with other agents in large hypertension trials and therefore, the doubt still remains as to whether β-blocker *monotherapy* can achieve reductions in mortality by virtue of its antihypertensive effect [6]. In terms of blood pressure reduction, the newer antihypertensive agents appear not to be superior to β-blockers such as atenolol [21].

The mechanism of action of β-blockers is shown in Fig. 12.3. Blood pressure reductions are proportional to the initial level. Falls by as much as 100/60 mmHg may occur in severe hypertension. Falls by 7–16/6–10 mmHg are characteristic of patients with mild hypertension. The blood pressure fall is greater in patients with high-renin hypertension.

β-Blockers have been shown to reduce the incidence of MI in non-diabetic, hypertensive men and women [22]. Furthermore, β-blockers reduce the incidence of MI, sudden death and all-cause mortality in survivors of MI [23–29]. In a recent retrospective study of 201 752 MI patients, treatment with β-blockers was associated with a 40% reduction in mortality at 2 years

[30]. Importantly, this benefit extended to patients with conditions that are often considered contra-indications to β-blockade (heart failure, chronic obstructive airways disease, diabetes mellitus, older age) and patients with non-Q wave MIs.

The cardioprotective effects of β-blockers may be linked to the antagonist effect of β-blockers on the pro-arrhythmic action of catecholamines — an effect which raises the threshold for ventricular fibrillation. Ventricular tachy-arrythmias are not uncommon in hypertensive patients and, therefore, their anti-arrhythmic properties make them ideal agents in hypertensive patients with CHD. The reduction in heart rate produced by β-blockers is dependent on the degree of background sympathetic stimulation, which is maximal during exercise and minimal during sleep. A reduction in the velocity of cardiac contraction and cardiac oxygen consumption, and a prolongation of diastole increases coronary perfusion in patients with angina [31].

The different effects of β-blockers result from three pharmacological properties:

Cardioselectivity: Differences in the relative capacity of β-blockers to block β_1 and β_2 adrenoceptors partly determine this property. Selectivity for β_1 and β_2 receptors diminishes as the dose of β-blocker is increased. In addition, up to 35% of β-adrenoceptors in the heart are of the β_2 variety. Therefore, selectivity for β_1 and β_2 receptors should not be equated with cardioselectivity. Propranolol is regarded as β-non-selective, whereas atenolol and bisoprolol are regarded as relatively β_1-selective.

Intrinsic sympathomimetic activity (ISA): Some β-blockers act as both agonists and antagonists of the β-adrenoceptors. Background sympathetic tone modulates this balance: the higher the sympathetic tone, the less the agonism; the lower the sympathetic tone, the more the agonism. Agents with a high ISA are less effective in reducing heart rate, which may even increase at night. Thus, β-blockers with a low or no ISA are preferred in hypertension, particularly in situations of increased sympathetic drive, such as stress, or in patients with exercise-induced tachyarrhythmias. Increasing ISA is associated with fine tremor and muscle cramps (with raised creatine kinase levels), although it gives rise to less fatigue, cold peripheries and metabolic disturbances.

Other properties: Labetolol and carvedilol have additional α-blocking properties that translate to a reduction in peripheral resistance. Such dual acting β-blockers have little effect on resting heart rate. The membrane stabilizing effect of propranolol, oxprenolol, labetalol and acebutolol at high doses is not desirable in the treatment of essential hypertension. Hydrophilic agents that do not cross the blood–brain barrier, such as atenolol, produce less neurological side-effects. Sotalol, which has amiodarone-like (class III anti-arrhythmic) properties, should not be used in the treatment of uncomplicated hypertension.

Cautions and adverse effects

Fatigue and lethargy. These are the most common, even with β_1-selective drugs without intrinsic sympathomimetic or vasodilatory activities. A reduction in physical activity is observed with all β-blockers.

Reduced psychomotor speed and alertness [32]. This may preclude their use in patients who drive heavy goods vehicles, those who work on scaffolding, as well as aircraft pilots and athletes. Subtle changes in mood and behaviour are also seen with the water-soluble β-blockers.

Worsening peripheral perfusion. This condition, arising from the reflex vasoconstrictive response to a reduced cardiac output, could theoretically produce lower limb claudication in patients with peripheral vascular disease. However, atenolol, propranolol and metoprolol have been shown *not* to reduce walking distance in patients with mild-to-moderate chronic intermittent claudication [33–35]. On this basis, therefore, mild-to-moderate peripheral vascular disease should not be considered as an absolute contraindication to β-blockade. Caution should be taken in patients with critical limb ischaemia.

Sleep disturbances and hallucinations. These occur with the lipid-soluble β-blockers, such as propranolol.

Impotence and sexual dysfunction. These occur less often than with thiazides, amounting to an excess of 0.2% over placebo.

Dyslipidaemia. Elevations in plasma triglycerides and reductions in plasma HDL-cholesterol [36,37] are most marked with non-selective β-blockers. The newer agents celiprolol and carvedilol, which have not been studied in clinical outcome trials of hypertensive individuals, reduce plasma triglycerides and raise plasma HDL-cholesterol levels.

Masking diabetic symptoms. The capacity of non-selective β-blockers to reduce the perception of hypoglycaemia (by blocking sympathetic activation) has been over-emphasized and is seldom a problem with β_1-selective agents. It is more of a problem with Type I diabetes than with Type II diabetes.

Bronchoconstriction. Whilst it is true that β-blockers cause bronchoconstriction in patients with asthma, this is not necessarily the case for those with chronic obstructive pulmonary disease [38]. Chronic obstructive pulmonary disease should not be considered an absolute contra-indication to β-blockade, particularly in view of the 40% reduction in 2-year mortality after MI which has also been shown in patients with this condition [30]. The use of a cardioselective drug, started under close clinical supervision, is advisable. If acute β-blockade is necessary, as in acute MI, esmolol, an ultra-short-acting β-blocker, should be considered as a trial.

Mild heart failure. β-Blockers have been used successfully in the treatment of mild heart failure. This requires close specialist supervision.

Pregnancy. β-Blockers may cause intra-uterine growth retardation and fetal bradycardia and are probably best avoided in pregnancy, particularly after the second trimester.

Rashes and dry eyes. These occur rarely and are reversible on withdrawal.

Phaeochromocytoma. In this condition, β-blockers should only be used in combination with α-blockers.

Sick sinus syndrome. If β-blockers are to be used for the management of tachyarrhythmias in this condition, temporary cardiac pacing may be a necessary prophylactic measure to cover bradyarrhythmias.

Interactions
Marked bradycardia, second or third degree atrioventricular block in combination with verapamil and, uncommonly, with diltiazem. The untoward effects of β-blockers on glucose homeostasis, lipids and male potency are potentiated when used in combination with thiazide diuretics.

Absolute contra-indications
Severe heart failure; bradycardia of < 50 beats min^{-1}; second or third degree atrioventricular block. Intraventricular conduction defects, such as right or left bundle branch blocks, are not, in themselves, contra-indications to β-blockade.

Choice
There are over 70 different generic and proprietary products with different formulations, some of them in the form of combined formulations with diuretics or calcium channel blockers. In terms of efficacy and metabolic effects, $β_1$-selective β-blockers without ISA, such as atenolol or bisoprolol, are the most appropriate choice. Bisoprolol requires less attention to dose reduction in elderly patients or those with renal or hepatic dysfunction, as it possesses balanced renal and hepatic clearance.

Doses

In hypertension, doses need not be as high as previously used. Atenolol 50 mg o.d. is usually effective, but some patients may respond to 25 mg o.d. With bisoprolol, the antihypertensive effect is well sustained over 24 h at once-daily dosage of bisoprolol 5 mg o.d. This may be increased to a maximum of bisoprolol 20 mg o.d.

Follow-up

The antihypertensive effects of β-blockers are observed in a few days and the maximal effect occurs by 2–3 weeks. As with most antihypertensive agents, they should be stopped and replaced by an alternative drug if there is no hypotensive response. Sudden withdrawal may cause exacerbation of angina and therefore, a gradual reduction of dose is preferred. This should be done by changing to alternate-day therapy for a week, then stopping.

CALCIUM CHANNEL BLOCKERS

Effects

Although originally intended for the treatment of CHD, calcium channel blockers have gained popularity as antihypertensive agents. The long-acting agent nitrendipine [39] is the only calcium antagonist which has so far been shown to reduce mortality and morbidity in hypertensive patients. On balance, however, current evidence is not in favour of the use of short-acting calcium antagonists in the management of hypertension [40] (see under 'Cautions and adverse effects'). The mode of action of calcium channel blockers is shown in Fig. 12.4.

Cautions and adverse effects

Myocardial infarction. Short-acting calcium channel blockers at high doses have recently been linked to an increase in the incidence of MI [22] and mortality [41] in hypertensive patients, adding to earlier findings that nifedipine at high doses resulted in death when given to patients with unstable angina or MI [42]. These effects of high doses of short-acting calcium channel blockers have been linked to their adrenergic effects, negative inotropism, prohaemorrhagic and pro-ischaemic effects, their effects on platelet aggregation, and possible pro-arrhythmic effects [41]. The interpretation of these deleterious effects has been challenged [6,43]. Two recent studies comparing metoprolol to verapamil [44] and atenolol to nifedipine (slow-release) [45] detected no difference in subsequent fatal or non-fatal cardiovascular events with these treatments in patients with angina. Furthermore, the Syst-Eur trial detected no adverse effect of nitrendipine on the incidence of MI [39]. Until the results of ongoing clinical trials emerge (the INSIGHT, ACTION, ASCOT,

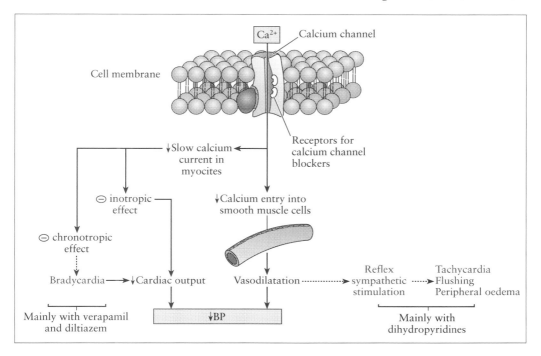

Figure 12.4 Mechanism of action of calcium channel blockers. Calcium channel bockers bind to the α_1-subunit of the calcium channel, causing a reduction in the influx of calcium into muscle cells. A reduction in calcium influx into the sarcoplasmic reticulum of smooth muscle cells leads to a reduction in smooth muscle contraction and resultant vasodilatation of peripheral and coronary arteries — their principal mode of action. Reductions in the slow calcium current in cardiomyocytes cause negatively inotropic and negatively chronotropic effects. A modest diuretic effect has been observed with dihydropyridines. The pharmacological effects of the various agents are determined by their chemical structure, lipophilicity and duration of action. The pharmacological subclasses are: the dihydropyridines (nifedipine, amlodipine, etc.); the benzothiazepines (diltiazem); and, the phenylalkalamines (verapamil).

ALLHAT studies), the use of short-acting calcium channel blockers, such as nifedipine, diltiazem and verapamil, in hypertensive patients, with or without CHD, must be discouraged [40].

Left ventricular dysfunction and heart failure. Calcium antagonists are generally contra-indicated in heart failure [46], although amlodipine appears to be safe [47].

Flushing, tremor, throbbing headache and sweating. These vasodilator side-effects, which occur in up to 30% of patients taking rapid-onset, short-acting dihydropyridines have been linked to reflex sympathetic nervous system activation and the rate of rise of blood dihydropyridine levels [48]. They are less often seen with slow-release preparations and the longer acting dihydropyridines, such as amlodipine. Vasodilator side-effects are not usually a feature of verapamil or diltiazem.

Oedema. This is a result of precapillary vasodilation and not of salt or water retention [49] or adrenergic activation. It is most frequently seen with the dihydropyridines and there is no suggestion that it is less common with longer-acting preparations (up to 30% with nifedipine 180 mg).

Constipation. This results from the reduction in gastro-intestinal motility that accompanies calcium antagonism in gastro-intestinal smooth muscle. It is most characteristic of verapamil, which may cause constipation in up to 30% of patients.

Bradyarrhythmias. Verapamil and, to a lesser degree, diltiazem can cause prolonged sinus arrest and disturbances of atrioventricular conduction in susceptible patients.

Pregnancy. Calcium channel blockers are best avoided in the first trimester of pregnancy, but may be considered a safe option in the second and third trimesters.

Gastro-intestinal haemorrhage. Diltiazem, verapamil and nifedipine have been linked to an increased risk of gastro-intestinal haemorrhage [50] in patients aged > 67 years. Until these findings are fully evaluated in randomized controlled trials, we recommend that caution be taken in prescribing short-acting calcium channel blockers in elderly patients who have a history of gastro-intestinal haemorrhage or who are taking non-steroidal anti-inflammatory agents. The Syst-Eur trial found no effects of nitrendipine on the risk of gastro-intestinal haemorrhage [39].

Depression and suicide. Limited evidence from observational studies suggests that calcium channel blockers may increase the risk of depression [51] and suicide [40,52]. These findings require further evaluation, but for now the use of calcium antagonists should be reconsidered in patients who develop depression whilst on these agents.

Gum hyperplasia and erythema multiforme. The former is uncommon. The latter occurs rarely.

Interactions
As with other antihypertensive agents, the hypotensive effect of calcium channel blockers is increased when used in combination with another anti-

hypertensive agent. There is an increased risk of first-dose hypotensive effect when used with α-blockers. The combination of verapamil with β-blockers is notorious for causing prolonged sinus arrest and disturbances of atrioventricular conduction and should always be avoided. Combinations of β-blockers with diltiazem also lead to similar rhythm disturbances, but these occur less commonly.

Absolute contra-indications
First trimester of pregnancy; breast-feeding.

Choice
Over 35 different calcium channel blocker preparations are currently available worldwide. Diltiazem and verapamil are free of sympathetically mediated side-effects, but they may precipitate an MI in hypertensive patients [22]. Furthermore, their negative chronotropic effects may preclude the future addition of a β-blocker. The short-acting nifedipine at high doses has also been implicated in increasing the risk of MI in hypertensive patients [22,41]. Long-acting dihydropyridines such as amlodipine and nitrendipine are preferred if antihypertensive treatment with calcium antagonists is deemed necessary.

Doses
In adults, amlodipine should be commenced at 5 mg o.d. In the elderly, it is best commenced at 2.5 mg o.d. Nitrendipine can be started at 10 mg at night, progressing to a maximum of 20 mg b.d.

Follow-up
Doses can be doubled every 3 weeks until the effective tolerated dose is reached.

ANGIOTENSIN-CONVERTING ENZYME (ACE) INHIBITORS

Effects
ACE inhibitors are as effective in lowering blood pressure as diuretics and β-blockers (see Fig. 12.5). The ability of ACE inhibitors to reduce mortality and morbidity in patients with heart failure from CHD [53] is an important aspect of management in hypertensive patients. So far, captopril, ramipril, enalapril, lisinopril, zofenopril, quinapril and trandolapril have been shown to reduce morbidity and mortality in patients with heart failure.

ACE inhibitors have also been shown to reduce micro-albuminuria and prevent deterioration in renal function in diabetic [54–57] and non-diabetic [58–60] hypertensive patients. The risk of death and the need for dialysis or

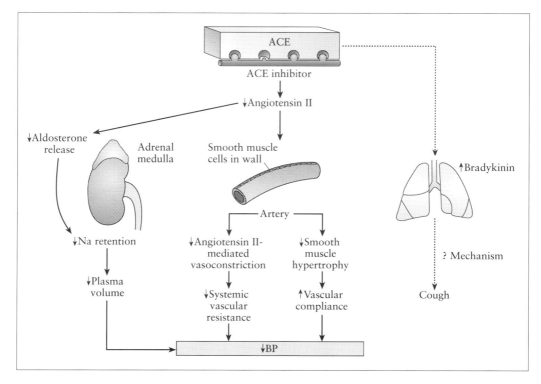

Figure 12.5 Mechanism of action of angiotensin-converting enzyme (ACE) inhibitors. ACE inhibitors exert their antihypertensive effects by competitively inhibiting ACE, which converts angiotensin I to the powerful vasoconstrictor angiotensin II. Reductions in the release of angiotensin II lead to a reduction in vascular tone and a decrease in circulating aldosterone. In addition, ACE inhibitors cause a reduction in systemic vascular resistance without changes in cardiac output or reflex sympathetic activation. Through reducing glomerular pressure and mesangial cell expansion, ACE inhibitors reduce protein excretion and improve renal function. In addition, ACE inhibitors appear to cause accumulation of bradykinin and prostaglandins in the lung and this action has been implicated in the generation of cough.

kidney transplantation in patients with non-insulin-dependent diabetes mellitus can be reduced by one-half using captopril [61]. The renoprotective effects of ACE inhibitors extend to both diabetic [62] and non-diabetic [63] nephropathies. These renal effects, which appear to be independent of the blood pressure-lowering effect, are characteristic of most ACE inhibitors, i.e. it is a 'class effect'.

The additional effects of ACE inhibitors on retinopathy are receiving increasing attention. Preliminary data from the EUCLID study suggest that lisinopril may retard the progression of retinopathy in normotensive patients with type I diabetes mellitus and early or no renal disease [64]. Attention is also being focused on the ability of ACE inhibitors to improve insulin resist-

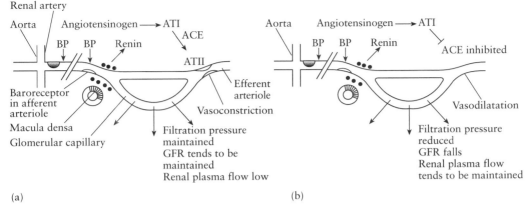

Figure 12.6 Mechanism of reduced glomerular filtration with angiotensin-converting enzyme (ACE) inhibitors. Renal haemodynamics (a) before and (b) after ACE inhibition. Adapted from [67].

ance [65], an apparent modulator of metabolic risk factors for cardiovascular disease [66]. Whilst these actions provide a potential for the use of ACE inhibitors in preventing and delaying end-organ damage, no clinical trials have addressed whether improving insulin resistance reduces mortality or morbidity in hypertensive patients nor, indeed, in any clinical situation.

Cautions and adverse effects

Dry cough. The commonest side-effect of all ACE inhibitors, cough, occurs in up to 15% of patients and it is more common in women. It does not respond to antitussives or non-steroidal anti-inflammatories. Because of its beneficial effects, however, treatment should not be automatically stopped. Some patients with heart failure feel so much better on ACE inhibitors that they are prepared to tolerate a dry cough (only about 4% of patients who suffer this side-effect actually discontinue treatment). If not tolerated, an angiotensin II (AT$_1$) receptor antagonist should be considered.

First-dose hypotension. This causes dizziness, lightheadedness, general weakness, visual disturbances, falling or syncope. Although some authorities favour hospitalization for all patients in whom ACE inhibitor therapy is to be initiated, this is impracticable in clinics. One should first stratify patients according to their risk of developing first-dose hypotension (Table 12.2) and then decide whether they should be supervised after administration of the first dose.

Table 12.2 Risk factors for first-dose hypotension with ACE inhibitor therapy.

Age > 70 years
Hyponatraemia (plasma Na < 130 mmol l^{-1})
Renal failure (plasma creatinine > 150 μmol l^{-1})
Renovascular hypertension
Renal artery stenosis*
Critical coronary artery stenoses
Heart failure requiring > 80 mg frusemide per day
Autonomic neuropathy (diabetes mellitus)

*Does not cause first-dose hypotension, but if present, may lead to acute renal failure. Patients with aortic aneurysm or intermittent claudication are more likely to have renovascular disease and therefore, are at an increased risk of renal failure with ACE inhibitors.

We suggest the following steps in the management of first-dose hypotension:

For patients at low risk:
- Prescribe a test dose of captopril 6.25 mg, to be taken at bedtime
- Instruct patients to report any adverse effects to the test dose before committing them to long-term therapy. These may be due to ACE effects, such as dizziness, lightheadedness and syncope; or dypsnoea, resulting from the rebound pulmonary oedema caused by diuretic withdrawal
- If no first-dose hypotension, continue on starting dose of ACE inhibitor plus usual medication
- Regardless of the ACE inhibitor chosen, measure serum creatinine within 5 days, and at 3 and 6 months of commencing therapy

For patients at high risk:
- Two days prior to test dose:
  - Check plasma electrolytes and creatinine
  - If taking a frusemide — equivalent dose < 40 mg day^{-1}: stop diuretics
  - If taking a frusemide — equivalent dose > 40 mg day^{-1}: halve the dose
- Administer a test dose of captopril 6.25 mg
- Monitor blood pressure every 15 min for 1 h and then every 30 min for 3 h
- Document *first-dose hypotension* if systolic blood pressure drops by > 40 mmHg. Beware of documenting dizziness, lightheadedness and syncope, or dypsnoea, resulting from the rebound pulmonary oedema caused by diuretic withdrawal
- If systolic blood pressure does not decrease by > 40 mmHg, start on the lowest dose of the chosen long-acting ACE inhibitor on the morning of the following day
- Regardless of the agent chosen, measure serum creatinine within 5 days, and at 3 and 6 months of commencing therapy

Renal artery stenosis. If bilateral, addition of ACE inhibitors can lead to deterioration of renal function within 24 h (Fig. 12.6) [67].

Hyperkalaemia. This is a theoretical risk. Out of 7402 patients treated with enalapril for 4–7 days in the SOLVD trial, one developed hyperkalaemia (the mean rise was 1.07 mmol l^{-1}).

Renal failure. The presence of renal failure is not a contra-indication to treatment with ACE inhibitors unless it is secondary to renal artery stenosis. Caution is required in using ACE inhibitors if the serum creatinine level is ≥ 200 µmol l^{-1} or if the serum potassium level is greater than 4.6 mmol l^{-1}.

Angio-oedema. This condition involving the face and limbs and, more ominously, the larynx, can occasionally occur. If it occurs, ACE inhibitors should not be used again.

Fever, serositis, myalgia arthralgia, a photosensitive skin rash. These conditions, together with a raised ESR and positive antinuclear antibody, have been described.

Pruritic rash. This is self-limiting.

A metallic taste. This is self-limiting.

Headache. This can also occur.

Fetal damage. All female patients of reproductive age must be warned of the risk of oligohydramnios and neonatal death from renal failure with ACE inhibitors [68]. If a hypertensive woman is contemplating pregnancy, ACE inhibitors should be substituted by non-teratogenic antihypertensive agents.

Interactions
As with other antihypertensive agents, ACE inhibitors enhance the hypotensive effects of other antihypertensive drugs. Severe postural hypotension may occur when combined with chlorpromazine, and possibly, other phenothiazines. Hyperkalaemia may occur when ACE inhibitors are combined with potassium-sparing diuretics, although this may not develop if loop diuretics are concurrently used.

Absolute contra-indications
These include known bilateral renal artery stenosis, haemodynamically significant aortic stenosis and pregnancy.

Choice

After adequate dose titration, ACE inhibitors are as effective as each other in lowering blood pressure. Generally, formulations containing active drugs act more rapidly than those containing prodrugs, but this is of little clinical value in long-term management. Agents with a long duration of action, which can be administered as a once-daily dosage are preferred. Fosinopril may offer advantages in the elderly because of its balanced renal and hepatic clearance, owing to compensatory excretion. Perindopril, at a dose of 2 mg orally, appears to be free of the first-dose response [69,70].

Follow-up

Generally, once first-dose hypotension has been addressed, ACE inhibitors can usually be titrated against blood pressure levels by doubling the dose until the highest tolerated dose is achieved. Maximal antihypertensive effects will occur in 2–3 weeks. Beware that a high, fixed dose of a long-acting ACE inhibitor in patients with heart failure may produce prolonged hypotension and end-organ ischaemia. There is no greater antihypertensive efficacy of one ACE inhibitor over another and therefore, there is little point in changing to another ACE inhibitor if the first one is not effective.

α-ADRENOCEPTOR ANTAGONISTS

Effects

The role of sympathetic overdrive and increased peripheral resistance in long-standing hypertension provides a theoretical rationale for blocking the stimulation of α-adrenoceptors (Fig. 12.7). Non-selective α-blockers, which act on α_1 and α_2 adrenoceptors, are no longer used. Selective α_1-blockers have not yet been shown to reduce morbidity or mortality in hypertensive patients, but this is currently being addressed in the ALLHAT trial [71].

Apart from their antihypertensive effects, α-blockers have an additional, beneficial effect on plasma lipids. Doxazosin has been shown to reduce total and LDL-cholesterol and triglycerides and to increase HDL-cholesterol in non-diabetic [72,73] and diabetic [74] individuals. Compared to thiazides and β-blockers, both prazosin [75] and doxazosin [73] are associated with a better lipid profile after 1 year of treatment. Small, non-controlled studies, have linked the beneficial lipid effects of α-blockers to their ability to reduce insulin levels and to improve insulin sensitivity [76]. The clinical significance of these effects on cardiovascular mortality and diabetic control or their perceived suitability in Asian and black patients with hypertension remains to be assessed.

Several randomized, double-blind trials have shown that doxazosin causes significant reductions in symptoms and increases in peak urinary flow rates [77]. Such changes occur at 2 weeks of treatment and reach a maximum after 7 weeks of treatment.

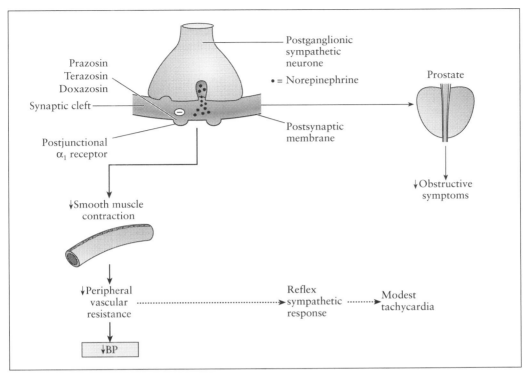

Figure 12.7 Mechanism of action of α-blockers. Selective α₁-blockers, such as prazosin, terazosin and doxazosin, exert their antihypertensive effects by reversibly inhibiting α-receptors post-junctionally, thereby causing relaxation of vascular smooth muscle and vasodilation. The lack of reflex tachycardia, such as occurs with other vasodilators, may be related to the ability of these drugs to reduce vascular tone in both resistance and capacitance vessels, or to a negative chronotropic effect. In addition to their antihypertensive effects, α₁-blockers also relieve the symptoms of prostatic obstruction by relaxing the bladder sphincter.

Cautions and adverse effects

First-dose hypotension. With prazosin, first-dose hypotension may occur in up to 40% of patients, culminating in postural syncope in up to 2%. This has not been extensively studied and therefore, we recommend that the same risk stratification and dose-titration measures are adopted for starting α-blockers as for starting ACE inhibitors (see p. 186).

Postural hypotension. Postural dizziness, which is dose related, occurs in 5–10% of patients, most often between 2 and 6 h after administration. All these symptoms can be minimized by close attention to dose titration. Whether doxazosin is less likely than prazosin to cause postural hypotension remains unresolved.

Other adverse effects. Fatigue, headache, nausea, palpitations and impotence are likely to occur in about 5% of patients. Impotence is less frequently seen with α-blockers than with β-blockers or thiazide diuretics. Withdrawal rates due to side-effects are about 5% for doxazosin.

Interactions

The hypotensive effects of α-blockers are enhanced by other concomitant antihypertensive treatment, particularly ACE inhibitors. Phenothiazines, levodopa, nitrates, hypnotics and anxiolytics also enhance the hypotensive effects of α-blockers. Non-steroidal anti-inflammatory drugs, pizotifen, tricyclics and corticosteroids antagonize their antihypertensive effect.

Choice

Prazosin has a relatively short half-life of 2–3 h and is therefore not suitable for long-term antihypertensive management. In contrast, doxazosin and terazosin can be administered as a once-daily dose, have a gradual onset of action, a more effective and predictable antihypertensive effect, and less side-effects than prazosin.

Doses

We recommend that with α-blockers, the same risk factors for first-dose hypotension as for ACE inhibitors are considered. To minimize the risk of postural hypotension, we recommend that doxazosin should be commenced at an initial dose of 1 mg day^{-1}. The dose can be doubled every 2 weeks to reach a maximum of 16 mg day^{-1}. Most patients can be maintained on doxazosin 2–4 mg o.d. Beyond 8 mg day^{-1}, there is no increased efficacy on benign prostatic hypertrophy. Terazosin is an effective antihypertensive at a dose of 2–10 mg o.d.

Follow-up

Response to initial treatment should be assessed at 2 weeks. Double the dose every 2 weeks thereafter, to reach a maximum dose of doxazosin of 16 mg day^{-1}. Dose adjustment is not required in renal dysfunction, but it is required in patients with hepatocellular damage.

ANGIOTENSIN II RECEPTOR ANTAGONISTS (ARAs)

Effects

The ARAs, such as losartan, valsartan, candesartan and irbesartan antagonize the hypertensive effects of the vasoconstrictor angiotensin II by blocking angiotensin II receptors (Fig. 12.8). Apart from being effective antihypertensive agents, ARAs may produce favourable effects on other aspects of hypertension, such as LVH, nephropathy and heart failure. Importantly,

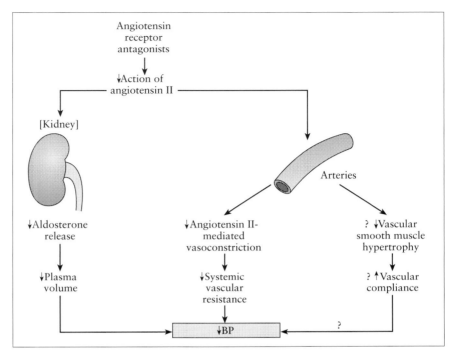

Figure 12.8 Mechanism of action of angiotensin II receptor antagonists (ARAs). Most of the known cardiovascular effects of the ARAs appear to be a result of their effects on the receptor subtype AT_1. In addition, the ARAs reduce noradrenaline release, stimulate the vasodilator prostacyclin, and counteract vascular wall hypertrophy. None of these mechanisms, however, have been satisfactorily assessed in humans and clinical outcome studies are necessary to ascertain whether these actions contribute to their clinical effects.

in the ELITE study of patients with heart failure aged > 65 years, treatment with losartan was associated with an unexpected lower mortality than that found with captopril [78]. A reduced frequency of cough, which may be due to a lack of effect of ARAs on bradykinin metabolism, offers an important and immediate advantage over ACE inhibitors. Some studies have shown that losartan has a uricosuric effect [79], causing a reduction in plasma uric acid levels [80]. The significance of this action is currently being addressed.

Cautions and adverse effects

Dizziness and orthostatic hypotension. These conditions may occur particularly during concomitant treatment with high-dose diuretics.

Hepatic and renal impairment. Dose adjustment is necessary.

Renal artery stenosis. The same cautions as for ACE inhibitors apply.

Hyperkalaemia. Plasma potassium levels should be monitored, particularly in the elderly and in those with renal impairment.

Absolute contra-indications
Pregnancy and breast-feeding.

COMBINATION THERAPY

In approximately 50 to 60% of patients, more than one agent is required to maintain blood pressure control [81,82] (Fig. 12.9). Generally, the greater blood pressure reductions required, the greater will be the need for the use of multiple agents [83]. As pointed out by Opie and Messerli in an elegant review [84], there are several reasons for combining antihypertensive treatment:
• It is combinations of antihypertensive drugs rather than monotherapy that have been used most frequently in the landmark studies of antihypertensive therapy showing a benefit in terms of mortality from stroke and CHD, e.g. β-blocker + thiazide diuretic was taken in 66% of patients in the STOP-Hypertension trial [85].
• Drugs in combination may have additive effects on blood pressure reduction, e.g. low-dose diuretics + β-blockers.
• Drugs in combination may exert complementary actions on specific end organs, e.g. verapamil + ACE inhibitor in reducing diabetic micro-albuminuria.

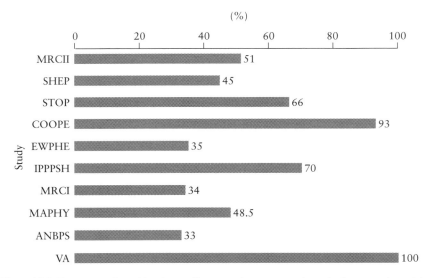

Figure 12.9 Frequency of combination antihypertensive treatment in major hypertension trials. Numbers denote the percentage of patients eventually requiring combination therapy despite the intention to treat with monotherapy. Reproduced from [14] with permission of Lippincott Williams & Wilkins, Philadelphia, PA.

• If different pharmacological classes are combined, one drug may counteract the adverse effects produced by the other drug, e.g. the reflex tachycardia produced by calcium antagonists is reduced by β-blockers.

• The use of lower doses in the combination may produce less dose-dependent side-effects than the drugs alone, e.g. metabolic side-effects of thiazides are reduced by combining them at low doses with ACE inhibitors.

FIXED-DOSE COMBINED FORMULATIONS

The ideal combined formulation should have the following properties:

• It should be superior to component drugs in achieving blood pressure control [86] and reducing or retarding the development of end-organ damage, such as LVH and renal failure.

• The component drugs should counteract each other's adverse effects.

• The component drugs must not interfere with each other, in terms of pharmacodynamics and pharmacokinetics.

• The formulation should give rise to less side-effects than the individual monotherapies.

• The cost of combined formulations should not exceed the cost of prescribing the individual drugs at the same dose.

In addition, because of the simplicity of use, they may improve long-term compliance. No studies have assessed whether fixed-dose combined formulations reduce mortality and morbidity in hypertensive patients. However, a large proportion of participants of the SHEP study [87], a study of isolated systolic hypertension, received chlorthalidone + atenolol and this combination was shown to reduce morbidity.

The following are some of the most commonly used combined formulations:

β-blocker + diuretic: Thiazides and β-blockers used in combination are more effective at reducing blood pressure than when the drugs are used alone. In addition, β-blockade counteracts diuretic-induced sympathetic nervous system activation and 'spares' diuretic-induced hypokalaemia. The combination of bisoprolol and hydrochlorothiazide, as well as achieving satisfactory blood pressure control, produces less side-effects than amlodipine or enalapril alone (bisoprolol and hydrochlorothiazide = 4%; amlodipine = 42%; enalapril = 47%) and withdrawal rates (4, 10, 14%, respectively) [88].

ACE inhibitor + diuretic: There are several theoretical reasons for combining these agents: ACE inhibitors produce reductions in the release of aldosterone, thus promoting potassium retention and counteracting the potassium loss produced by diuretics; the blood pressure lowering effect of diuretics is limited by reactive hyper-reninaemia, which is countered by ACE inhibitors; the sensitivity to ACE inhibition is increased by diuretics; and, the natriuresis produced by diuretics is promoted by ACE inhibitors. Numerous studies have shown that ACE inhibitors are more effective when combined with a diuretic [89–94]. Compared to component drugs, the combination is well tolerated, minimizes the incidence of diuretic-induced metabolic side-effects (hypokalaemia, glucose intolerance) and has a greater effect on left ventricular hypertrophy [95]. It should be considered that combined formulations of ACE inhibitors are also apt to cause first-dose hypotension and deterioration of renal function in susceptible patients. The use of test dosing (with captopril 6.25 mg) in susceptible patients is advised.

ACE inhibitor + calcium antagonist: This is an expensive combination, but it is well tolerated and effective at lowering blood pressure. Attention is currently being focused on the possibility that this combination may be particularly effective in retarding the progression of renal failure. Preliminary studies have shown that the combination of an ACE inhibitor with either verapamil or diltiazem in diabetics may be superior to monotherapy in retarding the progression of renal failure in diabetic patients [55,96]. More studies are needed to assess the role of the combination of ACE inhibitors + calcium antagonists in hypertension.

β-blocker + calcium antagonist: This combination generally improves antihypertensive efficacy without sacrificing tolerability. There are, however, no randomized controlled prospective outcome studies of this combination. Combinations of β-blocker and verapamil should not be used, because of the risk of asystole, bradycardia or hypotension.

β-blocker + ACE inhibitor: It is questionable whether this combination exerts an additive blood pressure lowering effect [97].

Combinations with α-blockers: Studies addressing combination of doxazosin with other antihypertensive agents involve small numbers of patients and no evidence-based recommendations can be made at present on this combination.

OTHER ANTIHYPERTENSIVE DRUGS

Loop diuretics

The loop diuretics, whose mechanism of action is shown in Fig. 12.2 (p. 172), are not recommended in the treatment of essential hypertension. They are less effective in the treatment of essential hypertension than the thiazides, produce a distressing diuresis and are more expensive. They are, however, more effective than thiazides in patients with renal impairment (glomerular filtration rate < 50 ml min^{-1}), fluid retention, heart failure and resistant hypertension. The potassium sparing diuretics (amiloride, triamterene and spironolactone) can be added to a thiazide or a loop diuretic to prevent hypokalaemia. This approach is more effective at preventing hypokalaemia than oral potassium supplementation.

Centrally acting drugs

Methyldopa. This reduces blood pressure by a central mechanism, probably involving depletion of noradrenaline and dopamine levels in the anterior hypothalamic–pre-optic region and in the medulla oblongata. Although not

Table 12.3 Doses of antihypertensive agents*.

Agent	Dose range (mg)	Frequency	Starting dose (mg)
Thiazide diuretics			
Bendrofluazide	2.5–7.5	o.d.	2.5
Hydrochlorothiazide	12.5–50	o.d.	12.5
Chlorthalidone	12.5–50	o.d.	12.5
β-Blockers			
Atenolol	50–100	o.d.	50
Bisoprolol	5–10	o.d.	5
ACE inhibitors			
Captopril (sulphydryl)	12.5–50	t.d.s.	test
Cilazapril	1–2.5	o.d.	test
Ramipril	2.5–10	o.d.	test
Enalapril	2.5–40	o.d./b.d.	test
Perindopril† (carboxyl)	2–8	o.d.	test?
Quinapril	10–40	o.d.	test
Trandolapril	1–4	o.d.	test
Lisinopril	2.5–40	o.d.	test
Fosinopril (phosphanyl)	10–40	o.d.	test?
Calcium antagonists (dihydropyridines)			
Amlodipine	5–10	o.d.	2.5
Lacidipine	2-6	o.d.	2
Nifedipine LA	30–90	o.d.	30
Felodipine	5–10	o.d.	5
α-Adrenoceptor blockers (β₁-selective)			
Doxazosin	2–32	o.d.	1
Terazosin	2–20	o.d.	1
Angiotensin receptor antagonists			
Losartan	50–100	o.d.	50
Candesartan	2–16	o.d.	2
Valsartan	80–160	o.d.	80
Irbesartan	75–300	o.d.	75
Combination therapy			
Enalapril + hydrochlorothiazide	20/12.5	o.d.	
Lisinopril + hydrochlorothiazide	10/12.5	o.d.	
Quinapril + hydrochlorothiazide	10/12.5	o.d.	
Atenolol + chlorthalidone	50/12.5	o.d.	
Atenolol + nifedipine	50/20	o.d./b.d.	

*Except for captopril, only agents with a long intrinsic duration of action are listed.
†Perindopril appears not to cause first-dose hypotension.

currently favoured in the treatment of essential hypertension, it is effective and safe as monotherapy and as an adjunct to other drugs [98,99]. In addition, it has no adverse effects on glucose, lipid and urate metabolism, nor does it adversely affect respiratory, renal and cardiac function. Methyldopa is the first choice drug for the treatment of hypertension in pregnancy (Chapter 9).

I_1-Imidazoline receptor agonists. The newly developed drug moxonidine lowers blood pressure by reducing sympathetic vasomotor drive centrally. It does this by acting on the I_1-imidazoline receptors in the rostral-ventrolateral medulla. Although moxonidine promises to be an effective antihypertensive agent, long-term outcome trials are required. The apparent effect on insulin sensitivity has only been evaluated in studies of small numbers of patients using surrogate measures. Further studies are needed to confirm this effect and to determine whether this might be favourable in patients with diabetes and/or other cardiovascular risk factors [100]. In combination with hydrochlorothiazide, moxonidine produces an additive hypotensive effect [101].

COST

Cost is an important consideration in antihypertensive management. Drug costs plus the cost of additional supervision and laboratory investigations should be balanced against the expected long-term benefit for a given patient. The issue of cost is particularly relevant in asymptomatic patients who have no end-organ damage or comorbid conditions. However, the preference for the cheapest drugs diminishes as the number and severity of co-existent conditions increases, as in these conditions the importance of the best drug becomes paramount.

References

1   Jones JK, Gorkin L, Lian JF, Staffa JA, Fletcher P. Discontinuation of and changes in treatment after start of new courses of antihypertensive drugs: a study of a United Kingdom population. *BMJ* 1995; 311: 293–295.
2   MRC Working Party. Medical Research Council Trial of treatment of hypertension in older adults: principal results. *BMJ* 1992; 304: 405–412.
3   SHEP Cooperative Research Group. Prevention of stroke by antihypertensive drug treatment in older persons with isolated systolic hypertension: final results of the Systolic Hypertension in the Elderly Program (SHEP). *JAMA* 1991; 265: 3255–3264.
4   Psaty BM, Furberg CD. Treatment trials: morbidity and mortality. In: Izzo JJ, Black H, Taubert K, eds. *Hypertension Primer: the Essentials of High Blood Pressure.* Dallas: American Heart Association, 1993: 197–201.
5   Thijs L, Fagard TR, Lijnen P *et al.* A meta-analysis of outcome trials in elderly hypertensives. *J Hypertens* 1992; 10: 1103–1109.

6 Opie LH, Messerli FH. Safety issues in combination therapy, with special reference to calcium antagonists. In: Opie L, Messerli F, eds. *Combination Drug Therapy for Hypertension.* New York: Lippincott-Raven Publishers, 1997: 158–173.

7 St John Hammond PG, Ratner P, Mullican W *et al.* Dose–response study of indapamide [abstract]. *J Am Soc Nephrol* 1993; 4: 451.

8 Fletcher AE. Adverse treatment effects in the trial of the European working party on high blood pressure in the elderly. *Am J Med* 1991; 90: 42S–43S.

9 Gurwitz JH, Kalish SC, Bohn RL *et al.* Thiazide diuretics and the initiation of anti-gout therapy. *J Clin Epidemiol* 1997; 50: 953–959.

10 Kasiske BL, Ma JZ, Kalil RSN, Louis TA. Effects of antihypertensive therapy on serum lipids. *Ann Intern Med* 1995; 122: 133–141.

11 Grimm RH Jr, Flack JM, Grandits GA *et al.* for the Treatment of Mild Hypertension Study (TOMHS) Research Group. Long-term effects on plasma lipids of diet and drugs to treat hypertension. *JAMA* 1996; 275: 1549–1556.

12 Neaton JD, Grimm AR, Prineas RJ *et al.* Treatment of mild hypertension study research group: final results. Treatment of Mild Hypertension Study. *JAMA* 1993; 270: 713–724.

13 Amery A, Birkenhager W, Bulpitt C *et al.* Influence of antihypertensive therapy on serum cholesterol in elderly hypertensive patients: Results of trial by the European Working Party on High Blood Pressure in the Elderly (EWPHE). *Acta Cardiol (Brux)* 1982; 37: 235–244.

14 Opie LH. Principles of combination therapy in hypertension. In: Opie L, Messerli F, eds. *Combination Drug Therapy for Hypertension.* New York: Lippincott-Raven Publishers, 1997: 1–10.

15 Carlsen JE, Kober L, Torp-Pedersen C, Johansen P. Relation between dose of bendrofluazide, antihypertensive effect, and adverse biochemical effects. *BMJ* 1990; 300: 975–978.

16 Siscovick DS, Raghunathum TE, Psaty BM. Diuretic therapy for hypertension and the risk of primary cardiac arrest. *N Engl J Med* 1995; 330: 1852–1857.

17 Law MR, Thompson SG, Wald NJ. Assessing the possible hazards of reducing serum cholesterol. *BMJ* 1994; 308: 373–379.

18 Antonios TF, Cappuccio FP, Markandu ND *et al.* A diuretic is more effective than a β-blocker in hypertensive patients not controlled on amlodipine and lisinopril. *Hypertension* 1996; 27: 1325–1328.

19 Singh BN, Hollenberg NK, Poole-Wilson PA, Robertson JIS. Diuretic-induced potassium and magnesium deficiency — relation to drug-induced Q-T prolongation, cardiac arrhythmias and sudden death. *J Hypertens* 1992; 10: 301–316.

20 Walma E, van Dooren C, Prins AD, van der Does E, Hoes A. Withdrawal of long term diuretic medication in the elderly: a double blind randomised trial. *BMJ* 1997; 315: 464–468.

21 Philipp T, Anlauf M, Distler A *et al.* Randomised, double blind, multicentre comparison of hydrochlorothiazide, atenolol, nitrendipine, and enalapril in antihypertensive treatment: results of the HANE study. *BMJ* 1997; 315: 154–159.

22 Psaty BM, Heckbert SR, Koepsell TD *et al.* The risk of myocardial infarction associated with antihypertensive agents. *JAMA* 1995; 274: 620–625.

23 Frishman WH, Furberg DC, Friedewald WT. β-Adrenergic blockade for survivors of acute myocardial infarction. *N Engl J Med* 1984; 310: 830–836.

24 Yusuf S, Wittes J, Friedman L. Overview of results of randomized clinical trials in heart disease: treatment following myocardial infarction. *JAMA* 1988; 260: 2088–2093.

25   Norwegian Multicentre Study Group. Timolol-induced reduction in mortality and reinfarction in patients surviving acute myocardial infarction. *N Engl J Med* 1981; 304: 801–807.

26   β-Blocker Heart Attack Trial Research Group. A randomized trial of propranolol in patients with acute myocardial infarction. I. Mortality results. *JAMA* 1982; 247: 1707–1714.

27   MIAMI Trial Research Group. Metoprolol in acute myocardial infarction (MIAMI). A randomized placebo-controlled international trial. *Eur Heart J* 1985; 6: 199–226.

28   ISIS-I (First International Study of Infarct Survival) Collaborative Group. Randomized trial of intravenous atenolol among 16 027 cases of suspected acute myocardial infarction. ISIS-I. *Lancet* 1986; ii: 57–66.

29   Roberts R, Rogers WJ, Mueller HS *et al.* Immediate versus deferred β-blockade following thrombolytic therapy in patients with acute myocardial infarction: results of the Thrombolysis In Acute Myocardial Infarction (TIMI) ii-B subgroup analysis. *Circulation* 1991; 83: 422–437.

30   Gottlieb SS, McCarter RJ, Vogel RA. Effect of β-blockade on mortality among high-risk and low-risk patients after myocardial infarction. *N Engl J Med* 1998; 339: 489–497.

31   Prichard BNC. Mechanisms of myocardial infarct prevention with β-adrenoceptor blocking drugs. *Drugs* 1983; 25 (Suppl. 2): 295–302.

32   Nerrick AL, Waller PC, Bern KE *et al.* Comparison of enalapril and atenolol in mild to moderate hypertension. *Am J Med* 1989; 86: 421–426.

33   Solomon SA, Ramsay LE, Yeo WW *et al.* β-Blockade and intermittent claudication: placebo-controlled comparison of atenolol and nifedipine and their combinations. *BMJ* 1991; 303: 1100–1104.

34   Bogaert MG, Clement DL. Lack of influence of propranolol and metoprolol on walking distance in patients with chronic intermittent claudication. *Eur Heart J* 1983; 4: 203–204.

35   Radack K, Deck C. β-Adrenergic blocker therapy does not worsen intermittent claudication in subjects with peripheral arterial disease. A meta-analysis of randomized controlled trials. *Arch Intern Med* 1991; 151: 1769–1776.

36   Weinberger MH. Antihypertensive therapy and lipids: evidence, mechanisms and implications. *Arch Intern Med* 1985; 145: 1102–1105.

37   Weinberger MH. Potential benefit of combination therapy with diuretics and β-blockers having intrinsic sympathomimetic activity. *Eur Heart J* 1990; 11: 560–565.

38   Woolcock AJ, Anderson SD, Peat JK. *et al.* Characteristics of bronchial hyperresponsiveness in chronic obstructive pulmonary disease and in asthma. *Am Rev Respir Dis* 1991; 143: 1438–1443.

39   Staessen JA, Fagard R, Thijs L *et al.* Morbidity and mortality in the placebo-controlled trial on isolated systolic hypertension in the elderly. *Lancet* 1997; 350: 757–764.

40   Stanton AV. Calcium channel blockers. The jury is still out on whether they cause heart attacks and suicide. *BMJ* 1998; 316: 1471–1473.

41   Furberg CD, Psaty BM, Meyer JV. Nifedipine: dose-related increase in mortality in patients with coronary heart disease. *Circulation* 1995; 92: 1326–1331.

42   Muller JE, Turi ZG, Pearl DG *et al.* Nifedipine and conventional therapy for unstable angina pectoris: a randomized, double-blind comparison. *Circulation* 1984; 69: 728–739.

43 Braun S, Boyko V, Behar S *et al.* Calcium antagonists and mortality in patients with coronary heart disease: a cohort study of 11,575 patients. *J Am Coll Cardiol* 1996; 28: 7–11.

44 Rehnqvist N, Hjemdahl P, Billing E *et al.* Effects of metoprolol vs verapamil in patients with stable angina pectoris. *Eur Heart J* 1996; 17: 76–81.

45 Fox KM, Muchany D, Findlay I, Ford I, Dargie HJ. Group on behalf of the TIBET Study. The Total Ischaemic Burden European Trial (TIBET). Effects of atenolol, nifedipine SR and their combination on the exercise test and the total ischaemic burden in 608 patients with stable angina. *Eur Heart J* 1996; 17: 96–103.

46 Elkayam U, Amin J, Mehra A *et al.* A prospective, randomized, double-blind, crossover study to compare the efficacy and safety of chronic nifedipine therapy with that of isosorbide dinitrate and their combination in the treatment of chronic congestive cardiac failure. *Circulation* 1990; 82: 1954–1961.

47 Packer M, Nicod P, Khandheria BR *et al.* Randomized, multicenter, double-blind, placebo-controlled evaluation of amlodipine in patients with mild-to-moderate heart failure. *J Am Coll Cardiol* 1991; 17: 274A [Abstract].

48 Kleinbloesem CH, van Brummelen P, Danhof M *et al.* Rate of increase in the plasma concentration of nifedipine as a major determinant of its hemodynamic effects in humans. *Clin Pharmacol Ther* 1987; 41: 26–30.

49 Gustafsson D. Microvascular mechanisms involved in calcium antagonist edema formation. *J Cardiovasc Pharmacol* 1987; 10 (Suppl. 1): S121–S131.

50 Pahor M, Guralnik JM, Furberg CD, Carbonin P, Havlik RJ. Risk of gastro-intestinal haemorrhage with calcium antagonists in hypertensive patients over 67 years old. *Lancet* 1996; 347: 1061–1065.

51 Hallas J. Evidence of depression by cardiovascular medication: a prescription sequence symmetry analysis. *Epidemiology* 1996; 7: 478–484.

52 Lindberg G, Bingefors K, Ranstam J, Råstam L, Melander A. Use of calcium channel blockers and risk of suicide: ecological findings confirmed in population based cohort study. *BMJ* 1998; 316: 741–745.

53 Latini R, Maggioni AP, Flather M, Sleight P, Tognoni G. ACE inhibitor use in patients with myocardial infarction. Summary of evidence from clinical trials. *Circulation* 1995; 95: 3132–3137.

54 Lewis EJ, Hunsicker LG, Bain RP, Rhode RD. The effect of angiotensin-converting enzyme-inhibition on diabetic nephropathy. *N Engl J Med* 1993; 329: 1456–1462.

55 Bakris GL. Effects of diltiazem or lisinopril on massive proteinuria associated with diabetes mellitus. *Ann Intern Med* 1990; 112: 701–702.

56 Bakris GL. Hypertension in diabetic patients: an overview of interventional studies to preserve renal function. *Am J Hypertens* 1993; 6: 140S–147S.

57 Makis DD, Ma JZ, Louis TA, Kasiske BL. Long-term effects of antihypertensive agents on proteinuria and renal function. *Arch Intern Med* 1995; 155: 1073–1080.

58 Kloke HJ, Wetzels JF, van Hamersvelt HW *et al.* Effects of nitrendipine and cilazapril on renal hemodynamics and albuminuria in hypertensive patients with chronic renal failure. *J Cardiovasc Pharmacol* 1990; 16: 924–930.

59 Kamper AL, Strandgaard S, Leyssac PP. Effect of enalapril on the progression of chronic renal failure. A randomized controlled trial. *Am J Hypertens* 1992; 5: 423–430.

60 Mann JF, Reisch C, Ritz E. Use of angiotensin-converting enzyme inhibitors for the preservation of kidney function. *Nephron* 1990; 55 (Suppl. 1): 38–44.

61 Weidmann P. Hypertension and diabetes. In: Kaplan N, ed. *Metabolic Aspects of Hypertension.* London: Science Press, 1994: 2.1–2.23.

62   Maschio G, Alberti D, Janin G *et al.* Effect of the ACE inhibitor benazepril on the progression of chronic renal insufficiency. *N Engl J Med* 1996; 334: 939–945.

63   Sihm I, Shroeder AP, Alkjaer C *et al.* Regression of media-to-lumen ratio of human subcutaneous arteries and LVH during treatment with an ACE inhibitor based regimen in hypertensive patients. *Am J Cardiol* 1995; 76: 38E–40E.

64   Chaturvedi N, Sjolie AK, Stephenson JM *et al.* Effect of lisinopril on progression of retinopathy in normotensive people with type 1 diabetes. The EUCLID Study Group. EURODIAB Controlled Trial of Lisinopril in Insulin-Dependent Diabetes Mellitus. *Lancet* 1998; 351: 28–31.

65   Paolisso G, Gambardella A, Verza M, O'Amore A, Sgambato S, Varricchio M. ACE inhibition improves insulin-sensitivity in aged insulin-resistant hypertensive patients. *J Hum Hypertens* 1992; 6: 175–179.

66   Reaven GM. Banting Lecture: role of insulin resistance in human disease. *Diabetes* 1988; 37: 1595–1607.

67   Wilkinson R. Renal and renovascular hypertension. In: Swales J, ed. *Textbook of Hypertension*. Oxford: Blackwell Scientific Publications, 1994: 831–857.

68   Hanssens M, Kierse MJNC, Vankelecom F, Van Assche FA. Fetal and neonatal effects of treatment with angiotensin-converting enzyme inhibitors in pregnancy. *Obstet Gynecol* 1991; 78: 128–135.

69   Reid JL, MacFadyen RJ, Squire IB, Lees KR. Angiotensin-converting enzyme inhibitors in heart failure: blood pressure changes after the first dose. *Am Heart J* 1993; 126: 794–797.

70   MacFadyen RJ, Lees KR, Reid JL. Differences in first dose response to angiotensin converting enzyme inhibition in congestive heart failure: a placebo controlled study. *Br Heart J* 1991; 66: 206–211.

71   Davis BR, Cutler JA, Gordon DJ *et al.* Rationale and design for the Antihypertensive and Lipid Lowering Treatment to prevent Heart Attack Trial (ALLHAT). *Am J Hypertens* 1996; 9: 342–360.

72   Ferrari P, Rosman J, Weidmann P. Antihypertensive agents, serum lipoproteins and glucose metabolism. *Am J Cardiol* 1991; 67: 26–35.

73   The Treatment of Mild Hypertension Research Group. The treatment of mild hypertension study. A randomized, placebo-controlled trial of nutritional-hygienic regimen with various drug monotherapies. *Arch Intern Med* 1991; 151: 1413–1423.

74   Lehtonen A and the Finnish Multicenter Study Group. Lowered levels of serum insulin, glucose and cholesterol in hypertensive patients during treatment with doxazosin. *Curr Ther Res* 1990; 47: 278–282.

75   Stamler R, Stamler J, Gosch FC *et al.* Initial antihypertensive drug therapy: a comparison of α-blocker (prazosin) and diuretic (hydrochlorothiazide). *Am J Med* 1989; 86 (Suppl. 1B): 24–27.

76   Pollare T, Lithell H, Selinus I *et al.* Application of prozosin in association with an increase in insulin sensitivity in obese patients with hypertension. *Diabetologia* 1988; 31: 415–420.

77   Fulton B, Wagstaff AJ, Sorkin EM. Doxazosin; an update of its clinical pharmacology and therapeutic applications in hypertension and benign prostatic hyperplasia. *Drugs* 1995; 49 (2): 295–320.

78   Pitt B, Segal R, Martinez FA *et al.* for the ELITE Study Investigators. Randomised trial of losartan versus captopril in patients over 65 with heart failure (Evaluation of Losartan in the Elderly Study, ELITE). *Lancet* 1997; 349: 747–752.

79   Kauffman RF, Beans JS, Zimmerman KM *et al.* Losartan, a new nonpeptide angiotensin II (Ang II) receptor antagonist, inhibits neointima formation following balloon injury to rat carotid arteries. *Life Sci* 1991; 49: 223–225.

80 Bui JD, Kimura B, Phillips MI. Losartan potassium, a nonpeptide antagonist of angiotensin II, chronically administered p.o. does not readily cross the blood–brain barrier. *Eur J Pharmacol* 1992; 219: 147–150.

81 James IM. Which antihypertensive? *Br J Clin Pract* 1990; 44: 102–105.

82 Townsend RR, Holland OB. Combination of converting enzyme inhibitor with diuretic for the treatment of hypertension. *Arch Intern Med* 1990; 150: 1175–1183.

83 Hansson L, Zanchetti A for the HOT Study Group. The Hypertension Optimal Treatment (HOT) study: patient characteristics, randomization, risk profiles, and early blood pressure results. *Blood Press* 1994; 3: 322–327.

84 Opie LH, Messerli FH. *Combination Drug Therapy for Hypertension.* New York: Lippincott-Raven Publishers, 1997.

85 Dahlöf B, Lindholm LH, Hansson L, Schersten B, Ekbom T, Wester PO. Morbidity and mortality in the Swedish Trial in Old Patients with Hypertension (STOP-Hypertension). *Lancet* 1991; 338: 1281–1285.

86 Messerli FH. Combination therapy in hypertension. *J Hum Hypertens* 1992; 6 (Suppl. 2): S19–S21.

87 Kostis J, Berge KG, Davis BR *et al.* Effect of atenolol and reserpine on selected events in SHEP. *Am Heart J* 1995; 130: 359–366.

88 Prisant ML, Weir MR, Papademetriou V, Weber MA, Adegbile IA. Low-dose drug combination therapy: an alternative first-line approach to hypertension treatment. *Am Heart J* 1995; 130: 359–366.

89 McGregor GA, Markandu ND, Banks RA *et al.* Captopril in essential hypertension; contrasting effects of adding hydrochlorothiazide or propranolol. *BMJ* 1982; 284: 693–696.

90 Vlasses PH, Roptmensch HH, Swanson BN *et al.* Comparative antihypertensive effects of enalapril maleate and hydrochlorothiazide, alone and in combination. *J Clin Pharmacol* 1983; 23: 227–233.

91 Thind GS, Mahaptra RK, Johnson A, Coleman RD. Low-dose captopril titration in patients with moderate-to-severe hypertension treated with diuretics. *Circulation* 1983; 67: 1340–1346.

92 Shapiro DL, Liss CL, Walker JF *et al.* Enalapril and hydrochlorothiazide as anti-hypertensive agents in the elderly. *J Cardiovasc Pharmacol* 1987; 10: S160–S162.

93 Kochar MS, Bolek G, Klabfleisch JH, Olzinski P. A 52 week comparison of lisinopril, hydrochlorothiazide and their combination in hypertension. *J Clin Pharmacol* 1987; 27: 373–377.

94 Brown CL, Blackhouse CI, Grippat JC, Santoni JP. The effect of perindopril and hydrochlorothiazide alone and in combination on blood pressure and on the renin-angiotensin system in hypertensive subjects. *Eur J Clin Pharmacol* 1990; 39: 327–332.

95 Pool JL, Gennari J, Goldstein R *et al.* Controlled multicentre study of antihypertensive effects of lisinopril, hydrochlorothiazide and lisinopril plus hydrochlorothiazide in the treatment of 394 patients with mild to moderate essential hypertension. *J Cardiovasc Pharmacol* 1987; 9: S36–S42.

96 Bakris GL, Williams B. Angiotensin converting enzyme inhibitors and calcium antagonists alone or combined: does the progression of diabetic renal disease differ? *J Hypertens* 1995; 13 (Suppl. 2): S95–S101.

97 Belz G. β-Blockers and ACE inhibitors. In: Opie L, Messerli F, eds. *Combination Drug Treatment for Hypertension.* New York: Lippincott-Raven Publishers, 1997: 77–90.

98 Redman CWG, Beilin LJ, Bonnar J. Treatment of hypertension in pregnancy with

methyldopa: blood pressure control and side effects. *Br J Obstet Gynaecol* 1977; 84: 419–426.

 99 Cockburn J, Moar VA, Ounsted M, Redman CWG. Final report of study on hypertension during pregnancy: effects of specific treatment on the growth and development of the children. *Lancet* 1982; i: 647–649.

100 Krentz AJ, Evans AJ. Selective imidazoline receptor agonists for metabolic syndrome. *Lancet* 1998; 351: 152–153.

101 Frei M, Küster L, Gardosch von Krosigk P-P, Koch H-F, Küppers H. Moxonidine and hydrochlorothiazide in combination: a synergistic antihypertensive effect. In: Papp J, Ollivier J-P, eds. *I1-Imidazoline-Receptor Agonists: a New Concept in Hypertension. The Imidazoline Receptor Agonist Moxonidine.* New York: Raven Press Ltd, 1994.

13: Tailoring Pharmacological Treatment

The ultimate aim in antihypertensive management is to prevent or delay death and/or disease. Therefore, treatment must be geared towards preventing or reversing end-organ damage. Traditionally, antihypertensive therapies have primarily been aimed at reducing blood pressure levels. It is now widely accepted, however, that lowering blood pressure should not be the only goal in the management of hypertension. This approach has emerged from the recognition that hypertension is part of a 'syndrome' of mutually supporting disturbances that contribute to cardiovascular risk [1–3]. Further support relates to the empirical observation that a hypertensive individual with a number of modest risk factors may be at considerably higher risk than an individual with the same blood pressure and with one very high risk factor [4,5] (Table 13.1).

In contrast to the 'stepped-care' approach (Fig. 13.1), tailoring treatment consists of designing and fitting a treatment that the patient will wear for a lifetime. At present, no antihypertensive agent is ideal for all patients and all clinical settings [8]. In this sense, there is no general 'first-line' treatment

Table 13.1 The synergistic effect of risk factors in five hypothetical patients with different risk factor profiles.

Risk factors	Patient 1	Patient 2	Patient 3	Patient 4	Patient 5
Cholesterol (mmol l^{-1})	8.0	8.0	8.0	8.0	8.0
Triglyceride (mmol l^{-1})	1.5	1.5	1.5	1.5	4.0
HDL-cholesterol (mmol l^{-1})	1.5	1.5	1.5	1.5	0.8
Systolic blood pressure (mmHg)	120	120	120	200	200
Family history < 60 years	–	+	+	+	+
Smoking	–	–	+	+	+
Angina	–	–	–	–	+
Diabetes	–	–	–	–	+
Absolute risk of MI from 50–59 years (%)	5	7	30	52	100

Absence (–) or presence (+) of risk factor. Absolute risk was calculated using Boehringer-Mannheim's 'Spirit-Plus' calculator[6], which employs an algorithm based on the PROCAM study for cardiovascular disease in German men and women. Adapted with permission from (7).

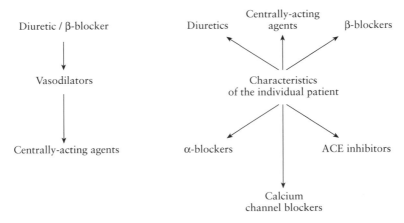

Figure 13.1 The stepped-care approach versus the tailored approach.

Table 13.2 Characteristics of hypertensive patients*.

	Men	Women
Age (years)	60 ± 10	64 ± 10
Blood pressure (mmHg)		
systolic	153 ± 17	156 ± 20
diastolic	91 ± 10	88 ± 10
Previous history of*(%):		
Myocardial infarction	8.3	2.8
Angina†	9.8	9.5
Diabetes mellitus	7.1	8.0
ECG-left ventricular hypertrophy	5.7	4.7
Valvular disease	5.4	8.2

*Patients with heart failure were excluded from the above. Analysis of 1128 men and 1374 women. The diagnosis of diabetes was defined on the basis of a fasting blood glucose of > 7.77 mmol l⁻¹ (140 mg dl⁻¹), two random non-fasting levels > 11.1 (200 mg dl⁻¹) or the use of insulin or oral hypoglycaemics. Results presented as mean SD or in the case of *, in %.
†With or without a previous myocardial infarction.
Adapted from [9].

of hypertension, despite the popularity of this term. In choosing the most appropriate drug, the clinician must start from the patient rather than from the drug or drug class. Hypertension frequently co-exists with related (Table 13.2) and unrelated conditions, all of which need to be taken into account when choosing antihypertensive drugs (Table 13.3).

Table 13.3 Considerations in evaluating hypertensive patients.

Age, sex, race and occupation.

Presence of hypertensive end-organ damage or conditions which are pathogenetically related to hypertension:
    Left ventricular hypertrophy
    Left ventricular dysfunction, symptomatic or asymptomatic
    Cardiac arrhythmias
    Renal damage, due to hypertension or other pathology
    Coronary heart disease
    Peripheral vascular disease
    Renal artery stenosis
    Aortic stenosis
    Diabetes mellitus
    Dyslipidaemia
    Gout
    Obesity

Presence of conditions which are pathogenetically *unrelated* to hypertension:
    Bronchoconstriction
    Prostatism
    Sexual dysfunction
    Sleep disturbance

Table 13.4 Classes of antihypertensive drugs.

Thiazide diuretics
β-Blockers
Calcium channel blockers
Angiotensin-converting enzyme inhibitors
Angiotensin II receptor-1 (AT_1) antagonists
Vasodilators
α-Blockers
Centrally-acting sympatholytics

TAILORING TREATMENT

Effectiveness at reducing blood pressure should not be a criterion in choosing drug classes (Table 13.4), given that drug classes have similar blood pressure-lowering efficacies in essential hypertension (Table 13.5). The following additional aspects may influence the choice of particular drugs.

Age

Most of the evidence on antihypertensive treatment in the elderly derives from studies of patients in the age range 65–80 years [11,12]. Large trials have convincingly demonstrated that elderly patients benefit from a reduction in blood pressure [13–15]. However, there is a general agreement that benefits diminish with increasing age [11,13–15] and that antihypertensive

Table 13.5 Comparative effects of different antihypertensive drugs*.

Treatment	Men	Women
Chlorthalidone (15 mg day^{-1})	−12.2	−12.5
Acebutolol (400 mg day^{-1})	−13.2	−12.9
Amlodipine (5 mg day^{-1})	−13.0	−12.8
Enalapril (5 mg day^{-1})	−11.7	−11.3
Doxazosin (2 mg day^{-1})	−11.7	−11.3
All drugs [+advice]†	−12.4	−12.2
Placebo [+advice]†	−9.1	−7.9

*Change in diastolic blood pressure (mmHg) over a 4-year period is shown. There is no significant difference in the blood pressure reduction achieved by the different agents. $P < 0.01$ for blood pressure reduction by all drugs compared to placebo.
†Note that patients receiving placebo, as well as those taking the active drugs, received advice on nutrition and lifestyle.
Adapted from [10].

treatment should only be considered up to the age of 75–80 [16]. No studies have specifically addressed whether antihypertensive treatment should be continued beyond the age of 80, but on the basis of circumstantial evidence, it seems prudent to continue treatment beyond this age in previously treated patients.

Isolated systolic hypertension is particularly common in the elderly and the evidence for the efficacy of thiazide diuretics in this group is overwhelming [15,17]. The SHEP study demonstrated that in patients > 60 years with isolated systolic hypertension, chlorthalidone 12.5 mg day^{-1} (as initial medication) reduced stroke incidence by 36% and CHD events by 32% over 5 years [12]. These findings are consistent with those of the Syst-Eur study [15], in which hydrochlorothiazide was the third-line trial drug. In another study of men and women aged 65–74 years, diuretics (hydrochlorothiazide 25 mg o.d. or 50 mg o.d.; amiloride 2.5 mg o.d. or 5 mg o.d.) were superior to β-blockers (atenolol 50 mg o.d.) at controlling blood pressure and reducing the risk of stroke and all cardiovascular events [11]. In the Syst-Eur study, treatment with the long-acting calcium antagonist nitrendipine led to a 42% reduction in fatal and non-fatal stroke over 2 years, although concomitant reductions in coronary events and heart failure did not reach statistical significance [15]. In view of these compelling findings, prescription in the elderly of more expensive antihypertensive agents should be resisted until further data on these agents emerge. The response to β-blockers in the elderly is less favourable than in young hypertensives [17,18].

Diuretic monotherapy, even at low doses, is not effective in young (< 60 years) white hypertensive male patients [19], but a good response has been observed in elderly male patients [12].

Preference

> 60 years: Low-dose thiazide diuretic, such as bendrofluazide 2.5 mg o.d.;
or chlorthalidone 12.5 mg o.d. increasing to 25 mg day^{-1}
< 60 years: β-blockers, such as atenolol 25–50 mg o.d.

It should be considered that withdrawal of long-term diuretic therapy in elderly patients can precipitate heart failure and therefore, careful monitoring is advised during the initial 4 weeks of withdrawal [20].

Race

Black people are more likely than white people to be hypertensive at all ages. In addition, black people are much more likely to die of stroke [21–23] and to develop end-stage renal failure [24]. As compared to the general USA population, hypertension in African-Americans develops at an earlier age, becomes more severe, and is associated with an 80% higher mortality from stroke, a 50% higher mortality from heart disease and a 320% greater rate of target-organ damage [25,26]. For these reasons, a more aggressive approach towards screening, follow-up and treatment of hypertension should be adopted in black patients. If hypertension is confirmed, the goal of antihypertensive treatment should be to keep blood pressure to ≤ 135/85 mmHg.

There is no ideal monotherapy for black patients with hypertension. ACE inhibitors are generally not effective as monotherapy, particularly in elderly black hypertensive patients. This lack of response has been linked to the greater incidence of low-renin hypertension in blacks. On the other hand, combinations of ACE inhibitors with low-dose thiazides does appear to be effective. Diuretics are generally considered to be more effective than β-blockers as monotherapy [12], although combinations of thiazides and β-blockers appear to be as effective in blacks as in whites. Calcium antagonists are as effective as hydrochlorothiazide and more effective than β-blockers or ACE inhibitors [27].

There are scarce data on antihypertensive treatment in Asian patients. Limited data suggest that they respond well to β-blockers [28–30].

Preference

Low-dose thiazide diuretics (bendrofluazide 2.5 mg o.d.) and long-acting calcium antagonists in black patients

Occupation

There are scarce data on the suitability of antihypertensive treatment in different occupations. β-Blockers may cause fatigue and postural dizziness and may adversely affect psychomotor speed, alertness [31] and intellectual activity. Although more characteristic of the lipid-soluble propranolol, such impairment has also been reported for atenolol at the usual doses of 50–100 mg day^{-1}. Such agents may therefore be considered unsuitable for patients who drive heavy goods vehicles, those who work on scaffolding, as well as aircraft pilots and athletes. On the other hand, β-blockers may be welcomed by those whose occupational activities cause anxiety. The choice of long-term treatment should perhaps be made after a trial period, having advised patients on possible psychomotor side-effects of β-blockers.

> ### Preference
>
> Consider avoiding β-blockers in occupations with a high physical and mental demand. For these occupations, one should consider angiotensin receptor antagonists given their substantially better side-effect profile.

LEFT VENTRICULAR HYPERTROPHY

Most antihypertensive agents, except for direct vasodilators such as hydralazine and minoxidil, reduce LVH [32]. In recent meta-analyses [33,34], ACE inhibitors appear to be superior to calcium antagonists, thiazide diuretics and β-blockers at reducing LVH. Whilst the results of these meta-analyses should be treated with caution (they are not direct comparisons of the effects of drugs), the recent RACE study of 193 patients has demonstrated that for the same reduction in blood pressure, left ventricular mass was reduced by ramipril, but not by atenolol [35]. Until prospective randomized, comparative trials address this issue, the presence of LVH should not automatically be regarded as an indication for treatment with ACE inhibitors. It is, however, prudent to consider ACE inhibitors in patients with LVH in whom there is, in addition, left ventricular dysfunction.

Further prospective randomized, comparative trials of sufficient size and duration are clearly needed. An important question that remains to be addressed is whether reversal of LVH confers benefits above those conferred by blood pressure lowering. In the meantime we recommend that ACE inhibitors be considered in patients with LVH. Their metabolic neutrality and their unsurpassed beneficial effects in patients with left ventricular dysfunction should also influence this decision.

HEART FAILURE AND LEFT VENTRICULAR DYSFUNCTION

No studies have assessed the impact on mortality of ACE inhibitors in patients with hypertensive heart failure. However, overwhelming evidence indicates that ACE inhibitors reduce mortality, delay the progression of ventricular dilatation and improve left ventricular dysfunction after acute MI (Chapter 12). So far, captopril, ramipril, enalapril, lisinopril, quinapril and trandolapril have been shown to reduce morbidity and mortality in patients with heart failure. On this basis, we recommend that ACE inhibitors be prescribed in all hypertensive patients who have had, *at any time*, signs of heart failure or left ventricular systolic dysfunction (ejection fraction of < 0.40 on echocardiography, radionuclide scans or LV angiography) (Chapter 5). In the ELITE study of patients with heart failure aged > 65 years, treatment with losartan was associated with an unexpected lower mortality than that found with captopril [36]. Further studies on the efficacy of angiotensin receptor antagonists in heart failure are awaited, but on the basis of the findings of the ELITE trial, losartan should be considered in patients with heart failure who develop a cough on ACE inhibitors.

β_1-Selective β-blockers reduce total and cardiovascular mortality and the incidence of non-fatal reinfarction in survivors of MI [37–43] — effects which may be related to their ability to improve cardiac function in the presence of ischaemia. α_1-Adrenoceptor blockers, with their capacity to reduce vascular tone in both arteries and veins offer theoretical advantages. Prazosin has been shown to produce significant reductions in systemic vascular resistance and an increase in stroke volume in heart failure, but it does not reduce mortality. Calcium antagonists do not improve mortality in heart failure. Short-acting agents, such as nifedipine, diltiazem and verapamil should be discouraged at present. The long-acting amlodipine appears to be safe [44]. It should be noted that the antihypertensive action of thiazide diuretics is impaired in the presence of left ventricular dysfunction.

> **Preference**
>
> ACE inhibitors
> The angiotensin receptor antagonist losartan in patients who develop a cough on an ACE inhibitor
> Combination of hydralazine and isosorbide dinitrate can be considered as alternative therapy if ACE inhibitors are not tolerated

CARDIAC ARRHYTHMIAS

At present, no evidence-based recommendations can be made regarding the preferential use of particular antihypertensive drugs in patients with ventricular ectopy. Sustained ventricular arrhythmias are likely to carry a greater risk of death than hypertension *per se* and should be referred to a cardiologist. Both chronic and paroxysmal atrial fibrillation in hypertensive patients carry a risk of embolic stroke and anticoagulant treatment as well as anti-arrhythmic therapy should be considered (Chapter 5).

> **Preference**
>
> Seek cardiology opinion
> β-Blockers in symptomatic ventricular ectopy

ANGINA WITHOUT HEART FAILURE

Angina results from an imbalance between myocardial oxygen supply and demand. Increased sympathetic activity plays an important role in angina as well as hypertension. Therefore, as competitive inhibitors of β-adrenoceptors, β-blockers are the agents of first choice in hypertensive patients with angina [45]. In addition, β-blockers should be preferentially considered in survivors of MI, as they reduce the incidence of subsequent MI, sudden death and all-cause mortality [37–43]. These benefits amount to a 20% reduction in long-term mortality and a 34% reduction in sudden cardiac death.

Although traditionally regarded as a contra-indication to β-blocker therapy, stable heart failure and left ventricular dysfunction can now be regarded as an indication for treatment with β-blockers. β-Blocker therapy in heart failure appears promising, both in terms of symptom control and in reducing mortality [46–48].

Caution must be exercised in prescribing short-acting calcium antagonists, given emerging reports of increased incidence of MI [49] and mortality

[50,51] in hypertensive patients. However, if β-blockers are ineffective or contra-indicated, diltiazem or verapamil should be considered in patients with angina with an intact cardiac function, given their ability to modestly reduce cardiac events and mortality in patients with non-Q MI and MI with preserved left ventricular function [52].

Although prazosin can prevent coronary spasm, no studies have adequately explored the effects of α-blockers in angina. Thiazide diuretics are of no specific value in angina. Limited clinical data suggest that ACE inhibitors may have an anti-anginal effect without producing a reflex tachycardia or a reduction in myocardial contractility.

Preference

β-Blockers

AORTIC STENOSIS

ACE inhibitors should be avoided in patients with haemodynamically significant aortic stenosis (when the Doppler-derived peak transaortic gradient is ≈ 40 mmHg or above). A cardiology opinion should be sought if ACE inhibitors are considered paramount as antihypertensive treatment in patients with aortic stenosis.

RENAL ARTERY STENOSIS

The detection of renal artery stenosis in hypertension is important because:
• It may be the cause of hypertension;
• It may be amenable to correction by surgery or angioplasty;
• It may lead to acute renal failure during treatment with vasodilators, particularly ACE inhibitors.

The presence of renal artery stenosis should be suspected in hypertensive patients with diabetes mellitus or those with an aneurysmal aorta or intermittent claudication, particularly if there is evidence of renal impairment or renal artery bruits on examination. If the plasma creatinine is elevated at the initial visit or if it rises by > 20 mmol l^{-1} following administration of ACE inhibitors, patients should undergo specific investigation for renal artery stenosis (Chapter 10).

Although ACE inhibitors should be avoided in patients with known renal artery stenosis, the finding of renal impairment on the initial visit should not automatically be regarded as a contra-indication to ACE inhibitors. Indeed, ACE inhibitors improve renal outcome in both diabetic [53] and non-diabetic [54] nephropathies. The renal impairment caused by ACE inhibitors in patients with renal artery stenosis is usually reversible on withdrawal of the drug, but persistent renal failure requiring dialysis may occur [55]. β-Blockers are particularly effective in patients with renal artery stenosis and those on renal haemodialysis (high plasma renin activity).

OBESITY

No evidence-based recommendations can be made regarding the preference of antihypertensive agents in obesity. Obesity is often associated with sympathetic overactivity, diabetes, impaired glucose tolerance and hyperinsulinaemia [1]. Thus the ability of ACE inhibitors to reduce angiotensin II levels and to improve insulin sensitivity [56] would appear advantageous. Although they inhibit sympathetic activity, α-adrenoceptor blockers do not appear to affect adversely insulin sensitivity and plasma lipid levels. Calcium channel blockers also appear to be metabolically neutral. It must be noted, however, that the association of insulin resistance and hypertension may not be causal and no studies have explored whether improving insulin sensitivity reduces morbidity or mortality. There is some evidence to suggest that the lipophilic ACE inhibitor trandolapril is more effective than captopril at reducing diastolic pressure in obese subjects.

Preference
None at present

DYSLIPIDAEMIA

It has been suggested that the less than expected reduction in CHD observed in trials of thiazide diuretics and β-blockers may be attributable to the untoward metabolic effects of these drugs. In this respect, it is noteworthy that even a 1% reduction in total cholesterol produces detectable 1% change in all-cause mortality [57]. It has also been proposed that antihypertensive drugs that do not produce untoward metabolic side-effects, or that improve the lipid profile, may produce greater reductions in CHD. No studies have so far resolved this issue, but on the basis of current evidence, choosing a metabolically neutral antihypertensive drug in dyslipidaemic patients would seem prudent.

There is little doubt that *high-dose* thiazide diuretics induce short-term elevations in total plasma cholesterol, triglycerides and LDL-cholesterol [58]. These effects, however, are not produced by low-dose thiazide therapy [59]. β-Blockers have also been shown to increase triglycerides transiently and to reduce HDL-cholesterol levels [60]. In the background of these observations, it should be noted that, used either alone or in combination, thiazide diuretics reduce the risks of cerebrovascular and coronary events, regardless of whether lipid levels are normal or raised [61,62]. Likewise, β-blockers reduce overall mortality and recurrent MI in MI survivors [63], despite their 'untoward' lipid effects.

ACE inhibitors [58] and calcium antagonists do not adversely affect the lipid profile, whereas α_1-blockers reduce total and LDL-cholesterol and triglycerides and increase HDL-cholesterol [59]. Compared to thiazides and β-blockers, treatment with prazosin [64] or doxazosin [65] is associated with a better lipid profile, and this effect persists after 1 year of treatment. Doxazosin has also been shown to improve the lipid profile in patients with diabetes mellitus [66].

Preference

Avoid high-dose thiazide diuretics
Use simvastatin or pravastatin as specific lipid-lowering therapy
Doxazosin for patients with dyslipidaemia

DIABETES MELLITUS (TYPE II) AND INSULIN RESISTANCE

Although the UKPDS 39 has shown that the benefits of ACE inhibitors and β-blockers were similar in terms of macrovascular and microvascular outcomes in patients with type II diabetes [67], the recent CAPPP study showed that hypertensive patients treated with captopril-based therapy had a lower risk of developing diabetes than patients assigned diuretic or β-blocker-based therapy [68]. In two small studies, ACE inhibitors faired better than calcium antagonists in terms of reducing CHD events in diabetic patients [69,70]. ACE inhibitors should be used preferentially if there is evidence of left ventricular dysfunction [71].

The presence of diabetic nephropathy also warrants a preference for ACE inhibitors. These agents have been shown to reduce micro-albuminuria and prevent deterioration in renal function in diabetic [72–75] and non-diabetic [76–78] hypertensive patients. The risk of death, need for dialysis or kidney transplantation in patients with non-insulin dependent diabetes mellitus can be reduced by one-half using captopril [79]. These renal effects, which appear to be independent of the blood pressure-lowering effect, are characteristic of most ACE inhibitors, i.e. it is a 'class effect'.

α-Blockers and centrally acting agents should be used with caution in patients with autonomic neuropathy, whether or not they have orthostatic hypotension. Although calcium antagonists have a vasodilatory effect, they are less likely to cause postural hypotension in patients with autonomic neuropathy. Methyldopa and clonidine are notorious for causing orthostatic hypotension.

Insulin resistance is a feature of CHD, heart failure [80,81], hypertension, diabetes, obesity, hyperuricaemia and dyslipidaemia [1,3,82,83]. However, no data are available on what level of insulin sensitivity should be considered 'pathological' [84]. Furthermore, no studies have explored whether treatment of insulin resistance *per se* leads to a reduction in morbidity or mortality in hypertensive patients nor, indeed, in the context of any other disease.

Preference

Low-dose thiazide diuretics in type II diabetes mellitus
ACE inhibitors in patients with diabetes mellitus and proteinuria

---

GOUT AND HYPERURICAEMIA

Gout is associated with an increased risk of CHD, congestive cardiac failure and intracranial haemorrhage [85–87]. Although the epidemiology of hyperuricaemia is different to that of gout, hyperuricaemic individuals are at an increased risk of developing CHD [88]. Because of their hyperuricaemic effects, thiazide diuretics should be avoided in patients with a history of gout. Hyperuricaemia without previous gout or urate nephrolithiasis, however, should not be regarded as a contra-indication to treatment with thiazide diuretics. There is no evidence that elevations or reductions in serum uric acid levels observed during antihypertensive treatment have any bearing on clinical disease. Preliminary studies indicate that losartan has a uricosuric effect [89], causing a reduction in plasma uric acid levels [90]. The significance of this action is currently being addressed. Whether this effect is beneficial in patients with gout, CHD or heart failure has not been explored.

Preference

Avoid thiazide diuretics in patients with a history of gout or urate nephrolithiasis

---

RENAL FAILURE

Hypertension alone is responsible for approximately 28% of all cases of end-stage renal failure requiring dialysis [91]. Black people, the elderly (> 60 years) and patients with higher diastolic pressures are the groups of hyper-

tensive patients at greatest risk of chronic renal failure. Patients with pre-existing renal disease secondary to another condition, such as diabetes, are more likely to develop hypertensive renal disease. Whatever the cause may be, the detection of renal failure is important for several reasons:
- Its presence will dictate the choice of antihypertensive therapy;
- Some antihypertensive treatments may lead to further deterioration of renal function;
- Antihypertensive treatment may retard the progression or even reverse the development of renal damage diabetic and non-diabetic nephropathy.

There are little prospective data on the ideal blood pressure for the hypertensive patient with renal impairment. It appears that the rate of deterioration of renal function in patients with essential hypertension is independent of the blood pressure [92]. Limited retrospective data, however, suggest that blood pressure should be kept below 140/90 mmHg in hypertensive patients with renal impairment [92,93]. In hypertensive (non-diabetic) renal failure, ACE inhibitors appear to slow the progression to the end stage compared to β-blockers [94].

Preference

Avoid potassium-sparing diuretics
ACE inhibitors in patients with diabetic neuropathy or with proteinuria/micro-albuminuria

STROKE

Hypertension is the most common cause of strokes. The distinction between the aetiologically distinct types of strokes has not been made in large-scale studies of hypertension and therefore, uncertainty remains as to which is most susceptible to antihypertensive treatment. Notwithstanding, it is well established that antihypertensive treatment reduces the incidence of 'unclassified' strokes and transient ischaemic attacks [12].

Thiazide diuretics, β-blockers and the long-acting calcium antagonist nitrendipine have been shown to reduce mortality from stroke in hypertensive patients. There are no satisfactory clinical data on the effects of other antihypertensives on morbidity and mortality from stroke and no clinical studies have explored the impact of different antihypertensive treatments on the recurrence of stroke, i.e. secondary prevention of stroke.

Preference

Thiazide diuretics in combination with β-blockers

PERIPHERAL VASCULAR DISEASE

Atherosclerosis is a generalized disorder of the vasculature and accordingly, peripheral vascular disease is a common finding in patients with CHD or hypertension. Conversely, patients with overt [95] or occult [96–98] peripheral vascular disease are at a high risk of developing CHD. Almost all patients with peripheral vascular disease die from CHD. Therapeutic trials of antihypertensive treatment lack insufficient statistical power to ascertain whether blood pressure lowering leads to a reduction in peripheral vascular disease. Limited data suggest that antihypertensive treatment reduces mortality from dissecting aortic aneurysms [99].

Antihypertensive management in patients with peripheral vascular disease should follow the same lines as for those with CHD. β-Blockers, including β$_1$-selective agents, lead to a reflex vasoconstrictive response, which results in a reduction in peripheral perfusion. In well-designed clinical studies, however, atenolol, propranolol and metoprolol do not affect walking distance in patients with mild-to-moderate chronic intermittent claudication [100–102]. On this basis therefore, mild-to-moderate peripheral vascular disease should not be considered as a contra-indication to β-blockade. Caution, however, should be exercised in patients with critical limb ischaemia.

Note

β-Blockers are safe in patients with mild-to-moderate intermittent claudication

---

CONDITIONS UNRELATED TO HYPERTENSION

Prostatism

Over 25% of apparently well men over 40 years of age suffer from symptoms of benign prostatic obstruction, which may include poor stream, hesitancy, intermittent flow, postmicturition dribbling and sensation of incomplete bladder emptying. Irritative symptoms, related to abnormal bladder response to filling (detrusor instability) include nocturia, frequency, urgency and urge incontinence. In more than half of cases of benign prostatic obstruction, symptoms are likely to affect lifestyle [103].

The maintenance of smooth muscle is regulated by the sympathetic nervous system. Prostatic tissue is rich in α-adrenoceptors, which mediate smooth muscle contraction. α-Blockers decrease smooth muscle tone and urethral pressure, thus improving urinary flow rates and obstructive symptoms. Indeed, α-blockers are used specifically to treat prostatic symptoms. There are reports that, in this respect, they are more effective than finasteride.

Preference

The α-blocker doxazosin

Bronchoconstriction

β-Blockers are best avoided in patients with asthma. They need not, however, be automatically avoided in patients with chronic obstructive pulmonary disease, particularly if they have had an MI. In this respect, a recent retrospective study (201 752 patients) has shown that β-blockade was associated with a 40% reduction in mortality at 2 years after an MI [104]. This benefit extended to patients with chronic obstructive airways disease. The best approach is to employ a cardioselective agent. If β-blockade is needed acutely and worries exist with regard to bronchoconstriction, the use of esmolol (esmolol: i.v. infusion 100–300 μg kg^{-1} min^{-1}) is advisable. This is an ultra short-acting β-blocker whose effect quickly disappears on stopping the intravenous infusion.

Two small non-controlled studies of hypertensive patients with chronic obstructive airways disease [105,106] have shown that doxazosin does not affect lung function. Thiazides, ACE inhibitors, calcium antagonists and vasodilators are safe in bronchoconstrictive disorders.

Note

Avoid β-blockers in asthma and use cautiously in chronic obstructive pulmonary disease
All other antihypertensive drugs can be used as alternatives

Sexual dysfunction

Despite the large scale of recent trials on antihypertensive treatment, little information regarding male sexual function has emerged and even less information is available with regard to female sexual function. Nevertheless, it is diuretics that have most consistently been associated with impotence [107]. In the Medical Research Council Trial, bendrofluazide was associated with twice as many cases of impotence as those on placebo and for this reason, 2% of patients discontinued treatment [108]. Higher withdrawal rates of 5% have been reported with chlorthalidone [109]. In the Treatment of Mild Hypertension Study [110], patients taking chlorthalidone were more likely to develop erectile failure than those taking doxazosin (17% vs. 3%).

The association between sexual dysfunction and β-blockers, although frequently mentioned, has not been confidently established. Although α-blockers appear to be neutral or even improve sexual function, no evidence-based recommendations can be made in this respect. ACE inhibitors appear not to affect sexual function adversely. No data are available on calcium antagonists. It is often difficult to determine whether sexual dysfunction occurring in a hypertensive patient is due to the treatment. The clinical history should focus attention on whether sexual dysfunction preceded antihypertensive treatment.

Note

Sexual dysfunction may be more common with thiazides and β-blockers

---

ADDING OTHER DRUGS

In up to 60% of patients, more than one agent is required to maintain blood pressure control [111,112]. As a general rule, the greater blood pressure reductions required, the greater will be the need for the use of multiple agents [113]. If blood pressure is not controlled at follow-up, the following sequence should be considered in managing mild-to-moderate hypertension:
• Unless the first agent is a thiazide diuretic, increase the dose of the selected agent to the best tolerated dose;
• If there is no response to the first drug or the patient experiences side-effects, substitute the first drug with another drug of a different pharmacological class [114];
• If the patient tolerates the first drug but the response is not satisfactory, combine with a second drug that is known to have additive or synergistic effects on the first drug;
• If blood pressure is satisfactorily controlled on the combination of the two chosen drugs, try to withdraw the first drug [114];
• If blood pressure is not controlled on two drugs, consider the possibility of resistant hypertension or add a third drug of a different pharmacological drug class;
• If blood pressure is stabilized on two agents, consider fixed-dose formulations.

HYPERTENSION RESISTANT TO TREATMENT

Definitions of resistant hypertension vary widely. In the absence of satisfactory data, such definitions have inevitably referred to arbitrary criteria. The diagnosis of resistant hypertension should be made if blood pressure cannot be reduced to < 140/90 mmHg in patients who are adhering to an adequate and appropriate triple-drug regimen that includes a diuretic, with all three drugs prescribed at near maximal doses. The following aspects should be considered in cases of resistant hypertension:

• Poor compliance with drug or specific dosages, with non-pharmacological measures, or failure to return for follow-up. This may occur in ≈ 50% of patients;

• Concomitant use of drugs (prescribed or unprescribed) which reduce the effectiveness of antihypertensive drugs [non-steroidal anti-inflammatory drugs (NSAIDs) and oral contraceptives] or which increase blood pressure (corticosteroids, anabolic steroids, cyclosporin, erythropoietin, monoamine oxidase inhibitors, cocaine, *excessive* alcohol intake);

• White-coat effect;

• Pseudohypertension of the elderly;

• Use of an inappropriately sized cuff;

• Unrecognized or new cause of secondary hypertension — this is an extremely rare cause of resistant hypertension.

MANAGING COMPLIANCE AND SIDE-EFFECTS

Some patients may be tempted to think that failure to control their blood pressure relates to the doctor's lack of skill. It is incumbent on the clinician to explain the following general points:

• Antihypertensive treatment is unlikely to make them feel better;

• Monotherapy is effective in only ≈ 50% of cases;

• Once changed to a second drug, the likelihood of successful blood pressure control on that drug is generally ≈ 50%;

• The newer ('more sophisticated') drugs are not more effective in hypertension than the older drugs, such as thiazides and β-blockers;

• The newer drugs are as likely to be continued by patients as the older drugs (Table 13.6).

The appearance of side-effects is a common reason for patients discontinuing treatment of their own accord and thus, the management of side-effects becomes as important as managing hypertension *per se*. Side-effects may be

Table 13.6 Continuation rates for different antihypertensive drugs.

Drug class	Number of patients	3 months (%)	6 months (%)
Diuretics	12 157	52	41
β-Blockers	9 348	61	49
Calcium channel blockers	7 176	49	41
ACE inhibitors	5 811	55	45

Adapted with permission from [8].

Table 13.7 Dealing with side-effects.

	Try reducing dose if:	Change to other drug class if:
Thiazides	—	Hypokalaemia
β-Blockers	Bradycardia or postural hypotension	Bronchoconstriction
Calcium antagonists	Bradycardia or postural hypotension	Flushing or ankle oedema
ACE inhibitors	Postural hypotension	Dry cough, angio-oedema
Vasodilators	Persistent headache	—

dose-independent, such as cough and angio-oedema with ACE inhibitors, or dose-dependent, such as postural hypotension with all antihypertensives. In addition, side-effects may be transient, usually during commencement of therapy; or persistent, such as cough with ACE inhibitors (Table 13.7).

References

1 Kaplan NM. The deadly quartet: upper-body obesity, glucose intolerance, hyper-triglyceridemia, and hypertension. *Arch Intern Med* 1989; 149: 1514–1520.

2 Leyva F, Godsland IF, Worthington M, Walton C, Stevenson JC. Factors of the metabolic syndrome. Baseline interrelationships in the first follow-up cohort of the HDDRISC study (HDDRISC-1). *Arterioscl Thromb Vasc Biol* 1998; 18: 208–214.

3 Reaven GM. Banting Lecture: role of insulin resistance in human disease. *Diabetes* 1988; 37: 1595–1607.

4 Anderson KM, Wilson PWF, Odell PM, Kannel WB. An updated coronary risk profile: a statement for health professionals. *Circulation* 1991; 83: 356–362.

5 Kannel WB, Stokes J. Hypertension as a cardiovascular risk factor. In: Birkenhager W, Reid J, eds. *Handbook of Hypertension*, Vol. 6. Amsterdam: Elsevier, 1985: 15–34.

6 Spirit Plus Manual. The new infarct risk calculator. Mannheim: Boehringer-Mannheim, 1990.

7 Dunningham M. Multiple risk factors interact. *Costs and Options* 1997; 10–12.

8 Jones JK, Gorkin L, Lian JF, Staffa JA, Fletcher P. Discontinuation of and changes in treatment after start of new courses of antihypertensive drugs: a study of a United Kingdom population. *BMJ* 1995; 311: 293–295.

9 Levy E, Larson MG, Ramachandran SV, Kannel WB, Ho KKL. The progression from hypertension to congestive heart failure. *JAMA* 1996; 275: 1557–1562.

10 Lewis CE, Grandits GA, Flack J *et al.* Efficacy and tolerance of antihypertensive treatment in men and women with stage I diastolic hypertension: results of the Treatment of Mild Hypertension Study. *Arch Intern Med* 1996; 156: 377–385.

11 MRC Working Party. Medical Research Council Trial of treatment of hypertension in older adults: principal results. *BMJ* 1992; 304: 405–412.

12 SHEP Cooperative Research Group. Prevention of stroke by antihypertensive drug treatment in older persons with isolated systolic hypertension. Final results of the Systolic Hypertension in the Elderly Program. *JAMA* 1991; 265: 3255–3264.

13 Dahlöf B, Lindholm LH, Hansson L, Schersten B, Ekbom T, Wester PO. Morbidity and mortality in the Swedish Trial in Old Patients with Hypertension (STOP-Hypertension). *Lancet* 1991; 338: 1281–1285.

14 Amery A, Birkenhäger W, Brixko R *et al.* Mortality and morbidity results from the European Working Party on High blood pressure in the elderly trial. *Lancet* 1985; i: 1349–1354.

15 Staessen JA, Fagard R, Thijs L *et al.* Morbidity and mortality in the placebo-controlled trial on isolated systolic hypertension in the elderly. *Lancet* 1997; 350: 757–764.

16 Thijs L, Van Hoof R, Staessen J, Fagard R, Celis H, Amery A. Drug treatment of hypertension in the elderly. In: Swales J, ed. *Textbook of Hypertension*. Oxford: Blackwell Scientific Publications, 1994: 1186–1194.

17 Management Committee. Treatment of mild hypertension in the elderly. A study initiated and administered by the National Heart Foundation of Australia. *Med J Aust* 1981; 2: 398–402.

18 Buhler FR, Laragh JH, Vaughan ED, Brunner HR, Gavras H, Baer L. Antihypertensive action of propranolol. *Am J Cardiol* 1973; 32: 511–512.

19 Meterson BJ, Reda DJ, Cushman WC *et al.* Single-drug therapy for hypertension in men. A comparison of six antihypertensive agents with placebo. *N Engl J Med* 1993; 328: 914–921.

20 Walma E, van Dooren C, Prins AD, van der Does E, Hoes A. Withdrawal of long term diuretic medication in the elderly: a double blind randomized trial. *BMJ* 1997; 315: 464–468.

21 Howard G, Anderson R, Sorlie P, Andrews V, Backlund E, Burke GL. Ethnic differences in stroke mortality between non-Hispanic whites, Hispanic whites, and blacks: the National Longitudinal Mortality Study. *Stroke* 1994; 25: 2120–2125.

22 Wild S, McKeigue P. Cross-sectional analysis of mortality by country of birth in England and E Wales 1970–92. *BMJ* 1997; 31: 705–710.

23 Cruickshank JK. National history of blood pressure in black populations. In: Cruickshank J, Beevers D, eds. *Ethnic Factors in Health and Disease*, Vol. 13D. London: Butterworth Heinemann, 1989: 268–279.

24 Qualheim RE, Rostand SG, Kirk KA *et al.* Changing patterns of end-stage renal disease due to hypertension. *Am J Kid Dis* 1991; 18: 336–343.

25 Singh GK, Kochanek KD, MacDorman MF. Advance report of final mortality statistics, 1994. *Mon Vital Stat Rep* 1996; 45 (Suppl. 3): 1–76.

26 Klag MJ, Whelton PK, Randall BL, Neaton JD, Brancati FL, Stamler J. End-stage renal disease in African-American and white men. 16-Year MRFIT Findings. *JAMA* 1997; 277: 1293–1298.

27 Zing W, Ferguson RK, Vlasses PH. Calcium antagonists in elderly and black hypertensive patients. *Arch Intern Med* 1991; 151: 2154–2162.

28 Kulpati DDS, Kaushal SS, Verma N, Raheja SM, Raghu A. Atenolol in the treatment of hypertension. *Ind Heart J* 1984; 36: 379–383.

29 Cheah JS, Chia BL. Propranolol in the treatment of hypertension of Asians. *J Trop Med Hyg* 1974; 77: 150–154.

30 Tsukiyama H, Otsuka K, Higuma K. Effects of β-adrenoceptor antagonists on central haemodynamics in essential hypertension. *Br J Clin Pharmacol* 1982; 13: 269S–278S.

31 Nerrick AL, Waller PC, Bern KE *et al.* Comparison of enalapril and atenolol in mild to moderate hypertension. *Am J Med* 1989; 86: 421–426.

32 Devereux RB. Do antihypertensive drugs differ in their ability to regress left ventricular hypertrophy? *Circulation* 1997; 95: 1983–1985.

33 Dahlöf P, Pennert K, Hansson L. Reversal of left ventricular hypertrophy in hypertensive patients: a meta-analysis of 109 treatment studies. *Am J Hypertens* 1992; 5: 95–110.

34 Schmieder RE, Martus P, Klingbeil A. Reversal of left ventricular hypertrophy in essential hypertension — a metaanalysis of randomized double-blind studies. *JAMA* 1996; 275: 1507–1513.

35 Agabiti-Rosei E, Ambrosini E, Dal Palù C *et al.* on behalf of the RACE Study Group. ACE inhibitor ramipril is more effective than β-blocker atenolol in reducing left ventricular mass in hypertension. Results of the RACE (Ramipril Cardioprotective Evaluation) Study. *J Hypertens* 1995; 13: 1325–1335.

36 Pitt B, Segal R, Martinez FA *et al.* for the ELITE Study Investigators. Randomized trial of losartan versus captopril in patients over 65 with heart failure (Evaluation of Losartan in the Elderly Study, ELITE). *Lancet* 1997; 349: 747–752.

37 Frishman WH, Furberg DC, Friedewald WT. β-Adrenergic blockade for survivors of acute myocardial infarction. *N Engl J Med* 1984; 310: 830–836.

38 Yusuf S, Wittes J, Friedman L. Overview of results of randomized clinical trials in heart disease: treatment following myocardial infarction. *JAMA* 1988; 260: 2088–2093.

39 Norwegian Multicentre Study Group. Timolol-induced reduction in mortality and reinfarction in patients surviving acute myocardial infarction. *N Engl J Med* 1981; 304: 801–807.

40 β-Blocker Heart Attack Trial Research Group. A randomized trial of propranolol in patients with acute myocardial infarction. I. Mortality results. *JAMA* 1982; 247: 1707–1714.

41 MIAMI Trial Research Group. Metoprolol in acute myocardial infarction (MIAMI). A randomized placebo-controlled international trial. *Eur Heart J* 1985; 6: 199–226.

42 ISIS-I (First International Study of Infarct Survival) Collaborative Group. Randomized trial of intravenous atenolol among 16,027 cases of suspected acute myocardial infarction. ISIS-I. *Lancet* 1986; ii: 57–66.

43 Roberts R, Rogers WJ, Mueller HS *et al.* Immediate versus deferred β-blockade following thrombolytic therapy in patients with acute myocardial infarction: results of the Thrombolysis in Acute Myocardial Infarction (TIMI) ii-B subgroup analysis. *Circulation* 1991; 83: 422–437.

44 Packer M, Nicod P, Khandheria BR *et al.* Randomized, multicenter, double-blind, placebo-controlled evaluation of amlodipine in patients with mild-to-moderate heart failure. *J Am Coll Cardiol* 1991; 17: 274A [Abstract].

45 Prichard BNC. Mechanisms of myocardial infarct prevention with β-adrenoceptor blocking drugs. *Drugs* 1983; 25 (Suppl. 2): 295–302.

46 Doughty RN, Rodgers A, Sharpe N, MacMahon S. Effects of β-blocker therapy on mortality in patients with heart failure. *Eur Heart J* 1997; 18: 560–565.

47 Doughty RN, MacMahon S, Sharpe N. β-Blockers in heart failure: promising or proved? *J Am Coll Cardiol* 1997; 23: 814–821.

48 Pfeffer MA, Stevenson LW. Beta-adrenergic blockers and survival in heart failure. *N Engl J Med* 1996; 334: 1396–1397.

49 Psaty BM, Heckbert SR, Koepsell TD *et al.* the risk of myocardial infarction associated with antihypertensive agents. *JAMA* 1995; 274: 620–625.

50 Furberg CD, Psaty BM, Meyer JV. Nifedipine: dose-related increase in mortality in patients with coronary heart disease. *Circulation* 1995; 92: 1326–1331.

51 Muller JE, Turi ZG, Pearl DG *et al.* Nifedipine and conventional therapy for unstable angina pectoris: a randomized, double-blind comparison. *Circulation* 1984; 69: 728–739.

52 Ryan TJ, Anderson JL, Antman EM *et al.* ACC/AHA guidelines for the management of patients with acute myocardial infarction: a report of the American College

of Cardiology/American Heart Association Task Force on Practice Guidelines (Committee on Management of Acute Myocardial Infarction). *J Am Coll Cardiol* 1996; 28: 1328–1428.

53 Maschio G, Alberti D, Janin G *et al.* Effect of the ACE inhibitor benazepril on the progression of chronic renal insufficiency. *N Engl J Med* 1996; 334: 939–945.

54 Sihm I, Shroeder AP, Alkjaer C *et al.* Regression of media-to-lumen ratio of human subcutaneous arteries and LVH during treatment with an ACE inhibitor based regimen in hypertensive patients. *Am J Cardiol* 1995; 76: 38E–40E.

55 Kalra PA, Mamtora H, Holmes AM, Waldek S. Renovascular disease and renal complications of angiotensin converting-enzyme inhibitor therapy. *Quart J Med* 1990; 77: 1013–1018.

56 Paolisso G, Gambardella A, Verza M, O'Amore A, Sgambato S, Varricchio M. ACE inhibition improves insulin-sensitivity in aged insulin-resistant hypertensive patients. *J Hum Hypertens* 1992; 6: 175–179.

57 Law MR, Thompson SG, Wald NJ. Assessing the possible hazards of reducing serum cholesterol. *BMJ* 1994; 308: 373–379.

58 Kasiske BL, Ma JZ, Kalil RSN, Louis TA. Effects of antihypertensive therapy on serum lipids. *Ann Intern Med* 1995; 122: 133–141.

59 Grimm RH Jr, Flack JM, Grandits GA *et al.* for the Treatment of Mild Hypertension Study (TOMHS) Research Group. Long-term effects on plasma lipids of diet and drugs to treat hypertension. *JAMA* 1996; 275: 1549–1556.

60 Lind L, Pollare T, Berne C, Lithell H. Long-term metabolic effects of antihypertensive drugs. *Am Heart J* 1994; 128: 1177–1183.

61 Frost PH, Davis BR, Burlando AJ *et al.* for the Systolic Hypertension in the Elderly Research Group. Serum lipids and incidence of coronary heart disease: findings from the Systolic Hypertension in the Elderly Program (SHEP). *Circulation* 1996; 94: 2381–2388.

62 Curb JD, Maxwell MH, Schneider KA, Taylor JO, Shulman NB. Adverse effects of antihypertensive medications in the Hypertension Detection and Follow-up Program. *Prog Cardiovasc Dis* 1986; 29 (Suppl. 1): 73–88.

63 Yusuf S, Peto R, Lewis J, Collins R, Sleight P. Beta blockade during and after myocardial infarction: an overview of the randomized trials. *Prog Cardiovasc Dis* 1985; 27: 335–371.

64 Stamler R, Stamler J, Gosch FC *et al.* Initial antihypertensive drug therapy: a comparison of alpha-blocker (prazosin) and diuretic (hydrochlorothiazide). *Am J Med* 1989; 86 (Suppl. 1B): 24–27.

65 The Treatment of Mild Hypertension Research Group. The treatment of mild hypertension study. A randomized, placebo-controlled trial of nutritional-hygienic regimen with various drug monotherapies. *Arch Intern Med* 1991; 151: 1413–1423.

66 Lehtonen A and the Finnish Multicenter Study Group. Lowered levels of serum insulin, glucose and cholesterol in hypertensive patients during treatment with doxazosin. *Curr Ther Res* 1990; 47: 278–282.

67 UK Prospective Diabetes Study Group. Efficacy of atenolol and captopril in reducing risk of macrovascular and microvascular complications in type 2 diabetes: UKPDS 39. *BMJ* 1998; 317: 713–720.

68 Hansson L, Lindholm LH, Niskanen L *et al.* for the CAPPP Study Group. Principal results of the Captopril Prevention Project (CAPPP). *Lancet* (in press).

69 Tatti P, Pahor M, Byington RP *et al.* Outcome results of the Fosinopril versus Amlodipine Cardiovascular Events randomized Trial (FACET) in patients with hypertension and NIDDM. *Diabetes Care* 1998; 21: 597–603.

70   Estacio RO, Jeffers BW, Hiatt WR *et al*. The effect of nisoldipine as compared to enalapril on cardiovascular outcomes in patients with non-insulin-dependent diabetes and hypertension. *N Engl J Med* 1998; 338: 645–652.

71   Garg R, Yusuf S, for the Collaborative Group on ACE Inhibitor Trials. Overview of randomized trials of angiotensin-converting enzyme inhibitors on mortality and morbidity in patients with heart failure. *JAMA* 1995; 273: 1450–1456.

72   Lewis EJ, Hunsicker LG, Bain RP, Rhode RD. The effect of angiotensin-converting enzyme-inhibition on diabetic nephropathy. *N Engl J Med* 1993; 329: 1456–1462.

73   Bakris GL. Effects of diltiazem or lisinopril on massive proteinuria associated with diabetes mellitus. *Ann Intern Med* 1990; 112: 701–702.

74   Bakris GL. Hypertension in diabetic patients: an overview of interventional studies to preserve renal function. *Am J Hypertens* 1993; 6: 140S–147S.

75   Makis DD, Ma JZ, Louis TA, Kasiske BL. Long-term effects of antihypertensive agents on proteinuria and renal function. *Arch Intern Med* 1995; 155: 1073–1080.

76   Kloke HJ, Wetzels JF, van Hamersvelt HW *et al*. Effects of nitrendipine and cilazapril on renal hemodynamics and albuminuria in hypertensive patients with chronic renal failure. *J Cardiovasc Pharmacol* 1990; 16: 924–930.

77   Kamper AL, Strandgaard S, Leyssac PP. Effect of enalapril on the progression of chronic renal failure. A randomized controlled trial. *Am J Hypertens* 1992; 5: 423–430.

78   Mann JF, Reisch C, Ritz E. Use of angiotensin-converting enzyme inhibitors for the preservation of kidney function. *Nephron* 1990; 55 (Suppl. 1): 38–44.

79   Weidmann P. Hypertension and diabetes. In: Kaplan N, ed. *Metabolic Aspects of Hypertension*. London: Science Press, 1994: 2.1–2.23.

80   Swan JW, Anker SD, Walton C *et al*. Insulin resistance in chronic heart failure: relation to severity and etiology of heart failure. *J Am Coll Cardiol* 1997; 30: 527–532.

81   Leyva F, Anker SD, Swan J *et al*. Serum uric acid as an index of impaired oxidative metabolism in chronic heart failure. *Eur Heart J* 1997; 18: 858–865.

82   Taskinen M-R. Strategies for the diagnosis of the metabolic syndrome. *Curr Opin Lipidol* 1993; 4: 434–443.

83   Modan M, Halkin H, Karasik A, Lusky A. Elevated serum uric acid — a facet of hyperinsulinaemia. *Diabetologia* 1987; 30: 713–718.

84   Godsland IF, Stevenson JC. Insulin resistance: syndrome or tendency? *Lancet* 1995; 346: 100–103.

85   Lichenstein L, Scott HW, Levin MH. Pathologic changes in gout. *Am J Pathol* 1956; 32: 871–877.

86   Sokoloff J. Pathology of gout. *JAMA* 1965; 152: 1106–1111.

87   Hall AP, Barry PE, Dawber JR, McNamara PM. Epidemiology of gout and hyperuricemia. A long-term population study. *Am J Med* 1967; 42: 27–37.

88   Klein R, Klein BE, Omae T, Takeshita M, Hirota Y. The relationship of serum uric acid to hypertension and ischemic heart disease. *Arch Intern Med* 1973; 35: 173–178.

89   Kauffman RF, Beans JS, Zimmerman KM *et al*. Losartan, a new nonpeptide angiotensin II (Ang II) receptor antagonist, inhibits neointima formation following balloon injury to rat carotid arteries. *Life Sci* 1991; 49: 223–225.

90   Bui JD, Kimura B, Phillips MI. Losartan potassium, a nonpeptide antagonist of angiotensin II, chronically administered p.o. does not readily cross the blood–brain barrier. *Eur J Pharmacol* 1992; 219: 147–150.

91   Whelton PK, Perneger TV, Brancati FL *et al*. Epidemiology of blood pressure-related renal disease. *J Hypertens* 1992; 10 (Suppl. 7): S77–S84.

92 Rosansky SJ, Hoover DR, King L *et al*. The association of blood pressure levels and change in renal function in hypertensive and non-hypertensive subjects. *Arch Intern Med* 1990; 150: 2073–2076.

93 Brazy PC, Stead WW, Fitzwilliam JF. Progression of renal insufficiency: role of blood pressure. *Kidney Int* 1989; 35: 670–674.

94 Hannedouche T, Landais P, Goldfarb B *et al*. Randomized controlled trial of enalapril and β-blockers in non-diabetic chronic renal failure. *BMJ* 1994; 309: 833–837.

95 Criqui MH, Langer RD, Fronek A *et al*. Mortality over a period of 10 years in patients with peripheral arterial disease. *N Engl J Med* 1992; 326: 381–386.

96 Salonen JT, Salonen R. Ultrasonographically assessed carotid morphology and the risk of coronary heart disease. *Arterioscl Thromb* 1991; 11: 1245–1249.

97 Norris JW, Zhu CZ, Bornstein MD, Chambers BR. Vascular risks of asymptomatic carotid stenosis. *Stroke* 1991; 22: 1485–1490.

98 McKenna M, Wolfson S, Kuller L. The ratio of ankle and arm arterial pressure as an independent predictor of mortality. *Atherosclerosis* 1991; 87: 119–128.

99 Veterans Administration Cooperative Study Group on Antihypertensive Agents. Effects of treatment on morbidity in hypertension: results in patients with diastolic blood pressures averaging 115 through 129 mmHg. *JAMA* 1967; 202: 1028–1034.

100 Solomon SA, Ramsay LE, Yeo WW *et al*. β-Blockade and intermittent claudication: placebo-controlled comparison of atenolol and nifedipine and their combinations. *BMJ* 1991; 303: 1100–1104.

101 Bogaert MG, Clement DL. Lack of influence of propranolol and metoprolol on walking distance in patients with chronic intermittent claudication. *Eur Heart J* 1983; 4: 203–204.

102 Radack K, Deck C. β-Adrenergic blocker therapy does not worsen intermittent claudication in subjects with peripheral arterial disease. A meta-analysis of randomized controlled trials. *Arch Intern Med* 1991; 151: 1769–1776.

103 Garraway WM, Collins GN, Lee RJ. High prevalence of benign prostatic hypertrophy in the community. *Lancet* 1991; 338: 469–471.

104 Gottlieb SS, McCarter RJ, Vogel RA. Effect of β-blockade on mortality among high-risk and low-risk patients after myocardial infarction. *N Engl J Med* 1998; 339: 489–497.

105 Biernacki W, Flenley DC. Doxazosin, a new alpha-1-antagonist drug, controls hypertension without causing airways obstruction in asthma and COPD. *J Hum Hypertens* 1989; 3: 419–425.

106 Malerba M, Dotti A, Zulli R. Doxazosin in the treatment of hypertension in patients with chronic obstructive pulmonary disease. *Curr Ther Res* 1991; 50: 27–37.

107 Wassertheil-Smoller S, Oberman A, Blaufox MD *et al*. The Trial of Antihypertensive Interventions and Management (TAIM) Study. Final results with regard to blood pressure, cardiovascular risk, and quality of life. *Am J Hypertens* 1992; 5: 37–44.

108 Medical Research Council trial of treatment of hypertension in older adults. *BMJ* 1992; 204: 405–412.

109 Curb JD, Borhani NO, Blaszkanski RP, Simbaldi F, Williams W. Long-term surveillance for adverse effects of antihypertensive drugs. *JAMA* 1985; 253: 3263–3268.

110 Neaton JD, Grimm AR, Prineas RJ *et al*. Treatment of mild hypertension study research group: final results. Treatment of Mild Hypertension Study. *JAMA* 1993; 270: 713–724.

111 James IM. Which antihypertensive? *Br J Clin Pract* 1990; 44: 102–105.

112 Townsend RR, Holland OB. Combination of converting enzyme inhibitor with diuretic for the treatment of hypertension. *Arch Intern Med* 1990; 150: 1175–1183.

113 Hansson L, Zanchetti A and the Group for the HOT Study. The Hypertension Optimal Treatment (HOT) study: patient characteristics, randomization, risk profiles, and early blood pressure results. *Blood Press* 1994; 3: 322–327.

114 Materson BJ, Reda DJ, Preston RA *et al*. Response to a second single antihypertensive agent used as monotherapy for hypertension after failure of the initial drug. *Arch Intern Med* 1995; 155: 1757–1762.

Index